Thriving

with NEUROFIBROMATOSIS

Thriving with Neurofibromatosis
Copyright ©2010 Kristianne Hopkins

Printed version created 2010
Published by Perflexativity Press

247 Cypress Lane
Broomfield, CO 80020
rich@richhopkins.net
www.RichHopkins.com

Published in the United States of America

Editing, Layout, and Cover Design: Perflexativity Press
Cover Photo by Nikki Belyea - MoxieImages.com

Contents

Acknowledgements

I would like to thank my family and friends. You have helped me see things are more than they appear to be, and that fear does not have to be what leads you. Instead, it can be transmuted into a powerful energy that propels you to become more than you ever imagined.

Thank you to the National Institutes of Health (NIH), for listening to me and helping me realize that I am important, that my pain is real, and for actually treating my symptoms. Dr. Doug Stewart and Sarah Coombes, you are vital people in my daily journey to Thrive with NF.

Thank you to Make-A-Wish Foundations of Washington and Colorado. You helped me and my family realize that wishes and dreams DO come true. Even in the face of the scary and unpredictable paths of life, holding onto one's dreams can help them get through anything. You, too, are in the business of Thriving, not just through NF, but through so many obstacles life can create.

Special thanks to my husband, Rich. You have accepted all of me and continue to support my dreams and goals. Without you, this book would have never come to fruition. I am proud to be your wife, and look forward to spending forever with you. Thank you for loving me, bumps and all.

What is Neurofibromatosis?

Neurofibromatosis encompasses a set of distinct genetic disorders that cause tumors to grow along various types of nerves and, in addition, can affect the development of non-nervous tissues such as bones and skin. Neurofibromatosis causes tumors to grow anywhere on or in the body.

Types Of Neurofibromatosis

Neurofibromatosis (NF) has been classified into three distinct types: NF1, NF2 and Schwannomatosis.

Neurofibromatosis 1 (NF1): also known as von Recklinghausen NF or Peripheral NF. Occurring in 1:3,000 births, web characterized by multiple cafe-au-lait spots and neurofibromas on or under the skin. Enlargement and deformation of bones and curvature of the spine (scoliosis) may also occur. Occasionally, tumors may develop in the brain, on cranial nerves, or on the spinal cord. About 50% of people with NF also have learning disabilities.

Neurofibromatosis 2 (NF2): also known as Bilateral Acoustic NF (BAN), is much rarer occurring in 1:25,000 births. NF2 is characterized by multiple tumors on the cranial and spinal nerves, and by other lesions of the brain and spinal cord. Tumors affecting both of the auditory nerves are the hallmark. Hearing loss beginning in the teens or early twenties is generally the first symptom.

Schwannomatosis: a rare form of NF that has only recently been recognized and appears to affect around 1:40,000 individuals. It is less well understood than NF1 and NF2, and features may vary greatly between patients.

Source: Children's Tumor Foundation

Foreword

Neurofibromatosis type 1 (NF1) is one of the most, if not the most, common genetic disorders in humans. The first, best modern medical description dates to 1882 and was written by a German pathologist named Friedrich von Recklinghausen.

However, descriptions of NF1 go back hundreds, if not thousands of years. Some scholars have speculated that certain ancient Greek statues and Parthian coins depicted NF1!

Neurofibromatosis type 1 is famously associated with its namesake tumor, the neurofibroma. For a person living with NF1, one of them most difficult aspects of the disorder is uncertainty about the number of neurofibromas he or she will develop. Predicting tumor burden is an important and active area of research. Multiple café-au-lait macules (or birthmarks) are also seen on the skin of almost everyone with NF1. It is also important to realize that NF1 is associated with a long list of benign and malignant tumors, many of them rare.

In our image-oriented society, it is tough enough living with a disorder that so obviously affects one's appearance. In my experience studying NF1, however, I have learned that the "invisible" issues are equally challenging. These include problems with depression and anxiety, learning differences and lower self-esteem.

I think that Kristi does a wonderful job sharing her battles with some of these demons. Fortunately there are good treatments for these problems, once they are recognized. Since Kristi finished school there is now wider acknowledgment of (and resources for) the learning and attention problems that affect many children with NF1.

I have done my share of reading about and talking with people with NF1. Kristi's book offers a unique perspective on life with NF1 and is a real testimony to the challenges, and hope, that can come from living with (and tackling!) NF1. I expect this book will serve as an inspiration to many who really are struggling with NF1. Kristi may not have "the answers" for your particular situation, however she has certainly figured out a lot of questions in her own life. There is power to her story.

I once heard that "NF" stands for "not fun." This is no doubt true, and much work remains to be done to improve the lives of people with NF1. I cringe when I hear, all too often, stories from patients about cruel experiences with doctors who are plainly misinformed about NF1.

The general public needs to know about NF1. I occasionally get asked what disorder I study. When I say "neurofibromatosis" I see eyes glaze over by the time I get to "fibro." So I have learned to say, "I study a common genetic disorder that greatly increases the chance that adults and children develop tumors." Although longer, most people will at least ask a follow-up question or two, at which point I mention "neurofibromatosis."

Clearly, the world needs to know more about NF1. Consider the success that the autism and breast cancer communities have had in increasing the exposure and publicity of "their" diseases. This certainly could be done for NF1. "Thriving with Neurofibromatosis" is a solid first step in that direction.

Douglas R. Stewart, M.D.
Rockville, MD
December 2010

(*Editor's note:* Dr. Stewart received his M.D. from the University of Pennsylvania School of Medicine in 1998. He completed a residency in internal medicine at the Hospital of the University of Pennsylvania in 2001 and training in medical genetics at the Children's Hospital of Philadelphia in 2004. He is board-certified in both internal medicine and clinical genetics. His major research interests are the adult manifestations of RAS-pathway disorders (especially NF1 and Legius syndrome), next generation sequencing of NF1-associated tumors and the characterization of novel features of NF1.)

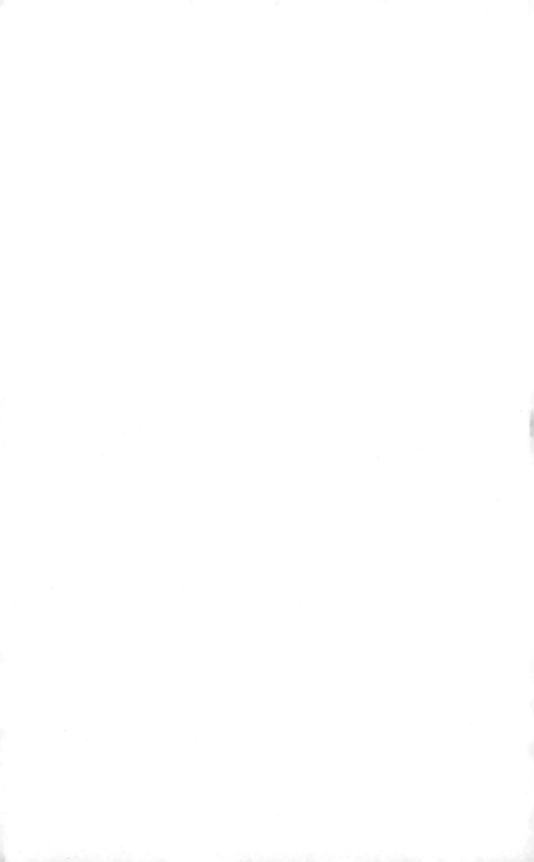

CHAPTER 1
Jump Ropes and Mud Puddles

I couldn't let them escape! I tied one end of my pink-handled jump rope around my waist, the other end around my older brother Jason. "Jay" and Kyle were always on the move, and I wanted to be sure they took me everywhere. I may have been dragging behind them, scraping up my knees and screaming, but I was happy to be a part of their lives any way I could.

I was the stereotypical pesky little sister, but my brothers didn't seem to mind me tagging along. They would frequently allow me to join in their Hot Wheels fun, digging dirt tunnels in our backyard. Whether it was playing with toy cars, climbing trees, or playing ball, I was a true Tomboy. I saw little advantage to being a dainty little girl.

I remember my brother's shock, when on a particularly hot California day, I dove into the mud bath we created in our backyard. Mom was yelling, "Don't get too messy Kristi!" But it was too late.

My brothers covered their faces, peeking through their fingers as I pretended the marvelous, muddy muck was a luxurious pile of bubbles, covering every inch of my body. My coolness factor spiked high that afternoon!

When Mom walked outside, my brothers slunk backwards, waiting for the inevitable explosion that builds inside parents of children determined to use mud as a fashion statement. She made her way toward me, her eyes opened wide, her hand over her mouth. But instead of anger, laughter burst out of her, as she began shaking her head in a combined look of disbelief and appreciation of my childhood spirit. Soon my brothers and I were splashing and sloshing in the mud as Mom looked on, exclaiming "Ohhh Kristi...Ohhh Kristi!"

We spent hours getting clean, using the cold blast of the water hose to wash away the multiple layers of mud, then hunched over the kitchen sink as Mom shampooed my hair over and over. She still couldn't stop laughing. Today she says she wishes she had taken pictures so that she could show Daddy.

Neurofibromatosis (NF) had no impact on me or how I lived my life before the age of seven. I didn't know I had it, and I barely understood that my brother Mike had it. I certainly didn't understand what he had gone through to that point, how it would transform my adult life, and affect the lives of my husband and six children.

But, it wasn't too long after our marvelous mud bath that NF began to wholly unravel my family.

I don't remember the reason, but on this particular night my brothers and I were camping in the living room, pretending to fall asleep to the TV. I was awakened by crying and sounds of convulsions, as Mike suddenly started throwing up. My mother was frantic, yelling at me to grab a bucket. Mike continued to get sick as Mom grabbed the phone.

"It's blood....I'm throwing up blood!" he yelled. It was everywhere. On the floor, on the couch. It looked like he'd been stabbed.

I just sat there staring. For the first time I realized how sick Mike really was. Jason and Kyle were running around with towels trying to help Mom clean Mike up. I was both stunned and terrified, and began to drift into my own little world.

Mike getting sick meant I was soon to be shipped off to my Aunt Pat and Uncle Ron. I loved their house, and never seemed to mind being away from my family. Probably because I became the center of attention, without any competition from my brothers!

Aunt Pat always had a cigarette in one hand, a Dr. Pepper in the other, and the best laugh I had ever heard. Some nights I would ask her why I was there, and she would very truthfully tell me that I was there because Mike was sick and needed Mom and Dad's full attention.

I slightly smiled at the thought of being able to go back with my Aunt, but was jolted back to reality when my mother slammed down the phone in a panic, "WHERE'S YOUR FATHER?!"

She ran over to my brother who was sitting on the couch, his head in the trash can. He was crying and shaking, telling Mom he was sorry for ruining the carpet. Washing off his face, she looked at Mike and told him that everything was going to be okay. Under her breath, I could hear her cursing my father for not letting her know where he was.

I was only six years old, but a gut-wrenching feeling came over me. While I couldn't know the world I lived in was about to be turned upside-down, I did know that things in my world weren't looking good.

I'm still not sure of the reason Mike got sick that night, though we believe it was a reaction to the chemotherapy he'd been going through to shrink a tumor he'd developed as a result of NF. I never went back to stay with my aunt and uncle. Instead, Mom and Dad decided to divorce.

It all happened so fast. I don't remember any conversations that prepared me for what was going to happen. I just remember being angry! I was mad at Mike for being sick. If only he could get better, we could be a family again. In my childhood mind, he was the reason Mom and Dad broke up. Real or not, my anger was reality for me.

To make matters worse, they split the family up. Mike and I went with Mom. For years, I felt like Mom got the 'defective' children - the sick kid and the dumb girl. I hated having to leave Dad, Kyle and Jay. I didn't want to go, but it didn't seem to matter to anyone but me. In what felt like an instant, my life was changed forever.

Try as I might, I just didn't have a jump-rope strong enough to keep my family together.

CHAPTER 2
Strong, Smart and Happy

After the divorce, Mom, Mike and I moved in with 'Dabbie', my Mom's Mom. She always said she wasn't old enough to be a grandmother, and never let us call her one. Dabbie had two major loves in her life: angel figurines and cigarettes. As much as I enjoyed looking at (and holding, when she wasn't around) the beautiful glass, crystal, and ceramic angels, I equally despised her cigarettes. I believe I cost her a large fortune in the few months we stayed with her from breaking, smashing, and otherwise destroying her stash of Winston's every chance I had.

As if dealing with the divorce and moving to a new home wasn't enough, I was put into a new school to start the third grade. On one hand, I hated starting a new school, on the other, no one here knew me. No one knew I'd been kept back in the second grade (something about me being overly social - can you imagine?). Mom told me the night before school began, "You can be anyone you want to be, Kristi. This is our fresh start." That advice has stayed with me my entire life.

I couldn't sleep the night before the first day of school. I started imagining who I could make myself into. Who could I be? I knew I wanted to be strong, smart, and most importantly, happy.

But being happy wasn't going to be easy. I was so angry at Mike for being sick. Nobody seemed to care about me. As a result, I had treated him like crap ever since the divorce, still blaming him for our family blowing apart. Inside though, I knew it wasn't his fault. I knew I was wrong to act the way I did. I suppose my first, somewhat accidental attempt to Thrive with NF (in this case, Mike's NF), began that night.

I smiled as I drifted off to sleep. Morning came, I dressed, stuffed a piece of toast down my throat and waited in the car – ready to be the new, stronger, smarter, and happier me.

Mom walked me to the school office, but I told her I wanted to go to class by myself. She left to take Mike to his new school, and I steeled myself for the grand entrance. Standing outside the door to my classroom, I licked my hands to slick my hair down. I straightened my shirt, briefly noticing a big brown stain. Ever the ragamuffin, my jeans came with holes and my shoelaces were forever untied.

Unconcerned about my fashion faux pas, I took a deep breath and repeated Mom's advice in my head: "You can be anyone you want to be." My tiny, trembling hand wrapped around the door knob and strained to open the heavy metal door. Slowly creaking the door open, I poked my head inside to look around the room.

Suddenly, with a surge of adolescent adrenaline, I pushed the door all the way open - smacking a poor brown-haired boy named Tommy right in the nose! He fell to the floor crying and holding his face, "My nose, my nose!" Blood dripped through his fingers as he scrambled to his feet and ran to the nurse's station.

I just stood there, twisting my feet and folding my arms. I bit my lip and handed the teacher the note from the office.

"Ahhh Kristi, our new student. Well...welcome to our class..." she sighed.

A few weeks later, it was here I experienced warning signs for Neurofibromatosis for the first time. The classroom started to spin. I fell out of my chair, and hit the floor hard. My classmates were laughing at me, and I couldn't get up. I felt sick to my stomach.

I looked up at the ceiling, feeling like I was on a boat. The rocking and swaying confused me, because I knew everyone around me was standing still. The teacher grabbed my arm and pulled me to my chair. I laid my head on my desk and shut my eyes. This was the first time I had ever experienced something like this, and it scared me. Fear doesn't last long in the young, of course, and when the dizziness finally stopped, I ran outside to join my friends on the playground.

Episodes like this were few and far between, but when they happened, calls home from the school went ignored. I felt like Mom didn't have time for another sick child, she worked too hard as it was. Now I realize that not only was she a single mom dealing with Mike's NF, which was continuing to have a negative effect on his quality of life, but she was also dealing with her own NF-related, deteriorating health.

For my part, I stayed quiet. I was not diagnosed with NF at this young age, and as far as mom was concerned I didn't have it, so she didn't have to worry. Even though the same doctor who had diagnosed my brother also examined me, and cafe au laits spots were noted, my parents were never told to follow up. As for my dizzy spells, they were repeatedly explained away, never linked to the disorder that coursed through my family tree.

The two years I spent in second grade ended up helping me a lot in third grade. I passed everyone up in my class, impressed my teachers, and was always asking for more work. The vision I had created for the 'new me' was coming true - I really was becoming stronger, smarter and happier.

The only exception came when I began to experience my first fears of having what Mike had. The school nurse was running routine lice checks, and her terse (and ignorant) assessment of my NF freckling consisted of "You're dirty – you need to wash your neck!" She gave me a note, and sent me on my way. Embarrassed, I ran home and jumped in the shower. I had no idea that I was dirty. I took baths every night, and I didn't smell bad.

I lathered up the soap between my fingers and washed my body. I took the scrub brush Mom used to clean the tub and went after the supposedly offending dirt. Now I was sure I was clean! But when I got out and looked in the mirror, I saw what the nurse was talking about. This "dirt" wasn't washing off. I got back into the bathtub and and let the water run over me. Scrubbing again I was determined to remove the 'dirt'. My neck quickly went from brown to red; from red to raw.

For the first time I felt different from everyone else, and I began to wonder if I could have NF too. I remember hiding the note from the school nurse, so Mom wouldn't read it. I didn't want to upset her more than she was.

Besides, I didn't need help. I was determined. I was strong, smart and happy.

No matter what.

CHAPTER 3
Bonnie and Clyde

That summer we moved out of Dabbie's house, and were excited to finally be moving into our own place. The cramped quarters of my grandmother's was beyond stressful. You could hear the eggshells cracking with every step. I loved my Dabbie, but she was an incredibly difficult person under even more difficult circumstances. Her primary coping mechanism seemed to be making my mother feel bad for every choice she'd ever made through the years. This was a trend that I, even at that young age, became determined to break.

We moved into a second floor apartment that sat along Roscoe Boulevard in Panorama City, California. The complex was right next to a drive-inn theater that proved easy to sit in on from the corner hillside, where Mike and I strained our ears to hear the speakers hanging from the car windows below. This was just a minor infraction, relatively, in what began a wild and crazy spree as we became our own juvenile versions of Bonnie and Clyde.

With Mom spending most of her waking hours at work, Mike and I had few boundaries. She had considered sending us both to a summer day camp, but it cost a fair amount of money to register. She was working hard just to make ends meet without creating another expense. Mike and I reassured her that everything would be fine – wink, wink!

Access to the apartment rooftops was literally child's play. We spent many afternoons entertaining ourselves by throwing eggs at the cars driving past below. Mom – now you know why we were always running out of eggs!

There were plenty of other kids in the complex, and we quickly made friends. Despite all the issues surrounding Mike and his NF, he was cool to hang out with. He was funny and always seemed to know his way around the city. Sometimes we'd get on the bus and just stay on it all day, laughing and joking until the bus driver finally had enough and ordered us off. Without Mike, I would have had no idea how to get back, so I was lucky to have him.

We were inseparable. As Mike was watching over me, I was watching over him. We protected each other. I made sure no one picked on or took advantage of him, and he always made sure I found my way home.

Mike made friends with everyone. With no money in our pockets, we often stopped at the local convenience store to swipe candy. Eventually, I got caught and Mike came to the rescue, getting me out of trouble because he knew the owner. Everywhere we went, someone knew him. It was amazing!

Some days, Mike would wear his Braille Olympics hat, bring along an old walking stick, and we would walk around collecting change for our lunch and bus fare. We pretended to be homeless! It was never hard to do, and people gave to us without hesitation. I don't know if we were that convincing or if they saw right through our pretend play and felt sorry for us. I still remember sitting at Winchell's Donut House counting our loot one day – three dollars and sixty-three cents! That was enough for a dozen donut holes, a soft drink, and a side trip to Bob's Market for my favorite: Nerds!

Our new home came with a pool right in the middle of the courtyard. When I wasn't busy being Bonnie, I was cementing my reputation as Krazy Kristi. It began innocently enough, as we watched Shannon, one of the older teenage boys, prove his manhood by jumping off the roof into the water below.

Full of bravado, he began taunting me: "Betchya too scared to do that!" While I was only nine years old, I wasn't going to let that go unpunished. I didn't go up to the roof, but I did climb over the second story railing, my arms holding tight the iron fence behind me, as I prepared to jump. Shannon was unimpressed. "You're not gonna do it! Chicken! Bawk Bawk!"

"Cowabunga!!!" I yelled as I jumped. With wild and joyful abandon, I hit the water hard, creating a terrific splash. "Ha!" I thought, "Betchya I'm NOT too scared!"

My younger self was never one to step away from a challenge, or avoid the spotlight. Later that summer, Mom took me to North Hollywood to try out to be a contestant on a new game show from Nickelodeon: DoubleDare. It wasn't on TV yet, and I had a chance to be one of the first people on it!

Bright and early Saturday morning, my mom drove Mike and me to the auditions. While you had to be between 8 and 12 to try out, Mike (who had just turned 14) went anyway to cheer me on.

The line of kids wrapped around the corner of the building. We stood waiting for two hours before I finally made my debut. Twelve other kids and I were told to run the obstacle course as fast as our bodies would move us. Best time wins.

I huffed and puffed my way through slime-filled slides, over ice cream-filled tires, and across whipped cream-covered floors. I didn't make the best time, but I had a ton of fun. I even caught a glimpse of dreamy Mark Summers, and I'm pretty sure he smiled and winked right at me!

I was interviewed after tryouts, for a potential role as a joke teller. I told the only joke I could remember:

A man calls up his house from work and a strange voice answers and says "hello"
"Who are you?" Says the man
"I'm the maid"
the man says "We don't have a maid!"
"Well, you know, your wife hired me today!"
So the man asks "What is my wife doing?"
The maid replies "She's in bed with her lover"
"IN BED WITH HER LOVER!??!" shouts the man
"Ok," the man says, "what I want you to do is go into the coat closet and get the shot gun and shoot my wife and her lover"
"Ok" the maid replies
She sets down the phone and the man hears two gun shots.
The maid comes back and picks up the phone
"Ok, I did it, now what?"
The man says "Take the bodies and throw them in the pool"
"Sir, what pool?"

The interviewers sat aghast for a few seconds. What did you expect from me, Krazy Kristi? A knock-knock joke? Needless to say, I didn't get the part.

Later that year, Mike was involved in a car accident. The door of the car he was in flew open, and he was thrown out. I was so scared of losing my brother, he was all I really had. Thankfully he wasn't seriously hurt, only breaking his shoulder blade. I wouldn't discover until later that Mike got a sizable settlement from that accident, which gave us a lot more financial flexibility for our adventures, and even MORE friends than he had before.

Mike would swipe the cash mom kept in her drawer, then wait until she had gone to work to wake me up for school. The first time Mike told me "Today, we're not going to school," I was a bit puzzled.

"Okay, but where are we going?" I asked.

We took the bus across town to the mall, playing in the arcade for hours, spending quarter after quarter on Pac-Man and Pole Position and stuffing ourselves with pizza - it was the greatest time - and best of all, Mom would never know!

Mike and I would do this a few times a month, until a phone call from my school prompted an investigation into why I was missing so much school. Tired and frustrated, my mother sat my brother and I down and, as you might suspect, screamed and yelled at us. "How can you do this? You know I have to work!" She was rightfully angry, but it went beyond anger, and for the first time, Mike and I were scared of Mom and the dark side that she was allowing to break through in a fit of fire and fury. It was all about what we were doing to her, and how awful we were making her life.

I was too young to truly understand what Mom was going through, but I did know that skipping school was never going to be fun again. Using the best little girl coping skills I had, I knew I had caused my mother pain and stress, something I never wanted to do, and from that moment on, I vowed to be the best daughter I could for my mom. I would make dinner, clean the house, and stay quiet - determined to get back on my mother's good side.

It didn't work.

With my brother's continued medical problems, my mother spiraled further into depression. She lost a lot of weight and seemed angry all the time. She worked long hours and her health noticeably suffered.

It was during this dark period that I first started to get an idea of what Neurofibromatosis was about. Mom and I shared her bed while Mike stayed down the hall in his room. I came in to the room one night just as she was putting on her bra, and noticed the bumpy skin on her back. I innocently asked "Mom, what are those bumps?"

She quickly covered up and her eyes filled with anger. "It's none of your business. They're just my bumps. God did this to me and your brother. God hates us." Scared, I asked if I would get them. "Probably. God hates us." she said again. That was the last time I would bring it up with her, until nearly 20 years later.

Mike's fight with NF was getting tougher. He began testosterone treatments because he was not entering into puberty. It appeared the radiation treatments that had blinded him in his right eye had also affected his pituitary gland in an irreversible and devastating way.

Testosterone brought out the beast in Mike. He became very aggressive, scaring me with his own sudden fits of anger, even putting a knife to my neck in a terrible rage. His pent-up anger directed itself at Mom as well, and while she did her best to deal with the changes her son was going through, it proved to be too much. She ended up breaking down, at times becoming abusive with Mike and I as she struggled with her own fear and pain.

A few weeks later, while sitting in the car waiting for my brother to come with me on visitation weekend with Dad, I confided in Susie (my dads fiancée) about my mom's struggles with Mike and me.

"Please don't tell my dad, but my mom got very angry the other day..." I went on to tell her that Mom had pushed me into the closet and told me she wished I'd never been born. Susie, of course, relayed this to my father, despite my plea. Little did I realize that it would initiate the process of my father taking Mike and I away.

The last time I saw Mom for the next several years was in the courtroom. She was standing against the wall as the decision was made to assign my father full custody. My brothers and I were playing bloody knuckles, and when I saw my mom walking out, she was crying and looking at me through her hands.

It all happened so fast, and I was confused. After thinking about it, what happened to me didn't seem that big of a deal – and I figured I probably deserved it. Besides, Mom would never mean to hurt me. I was sorry that I ever said anything to Susie. I wanted to hug my mom. I wanted to go with her. I saw how hurt she was, and it was all because of me. I looked at her, and I just wanted to run back into her arms and tell her I was sorry for being bad.

Dad made me and my brothers keep our distance, though. All I could do was raise my hand with my two middle fingers bent down, giving my mom the "I Love You" sign. She looked back at me and returned the gesture.

And then it was over.

CHAPTER 4
Little Orphan Kristi

Uprooted for my own safety, I had gone from one dysfunctional home to another. At ten years old, I just didn't know it yet. Dad and Susie did their best to help Mike and I make the transition. I got my own room with a beautiful new daybed, complete with an eyelet comforter. For the first time, I didn't have to share with anyone!

There was a large dresser and a large, empty closet. I remember hearing Susie tell my dad I looked like a 'ragamuffin' – and she was right. Mom had to shop at thrift stores, and my clothes were mostly jeans, sweats, and t-shirts. I didn't care much though. It was what I was used to, and frankly, they were pretty comfortable.

Susie wasn't a thrift store type. We headed out to the mall, and left with a new wardrobe of dresses, pleated pants, and designer shirts. I looked gooooood. She also took me out to replace my Barbies, which had been left at Mom's in the rush to get me out of her apartment. I felt sad and happy all at once. I was enjoying being with my dad and all my brothers again, as well as enjoying the reduced stress of my new living situation. Still missed my mom, and wondered if she was going to be okay without me.

Laying back on my bed, I thought about how nice it was to have such nice things, but then missed my mother terribly. I wondered who would take care of her. Wondered if she was laying in the bed we shared, thinking about me, and missing me too.

Dad and Susie's wedding was coming up, and Susie decided to take me out on a 'girl's only' errand to her hair salon. This would be my first real hair cut. My hair had grown down most of my back, without much maintenance, purpose, or style. I was excited about what a 'real, professional stylist' would do to me. I had visions of walking down the street with long, flowing, movie star hair, complete with steady wind blowing it back everywhere I went.

I sat high in the salon chair, straining to listen as Susie gave my stylist instructions on what superstar treatment I was to receive. As the woman ran her fingers through my hair, I just sat and smiled sweetly, content with my expectations. Suddenly, with a swift swipe of the scissors, my lifetime's effort of hair growing, nearly 8 inches of beautiful blond/brown hair dropped to the floor, shortly followed by my lower jaw.

Stunned, I was uncertain how to react. I didn't want to create a fuss, and I knew she couldn't exactly re-attach the piles of hair surrounding my chair. The stylist kept snipping, shaping my hair shorter...shorter...shorter...

Then she wheeled over a cart filled with curlers. I knew exactly what they were, because my mother had worn curlers in her hair every night. She tightly wrapped my hair, pouring that nasty, smelly stuff all over my head. The ensuing wait seemed like an eternity.

When the curlers were removed, and my hair was washed clean, the stylist turned me so I couldn't see the mirror while my hair was blown dry. Clearly, something was up. When my chair swiveled around, I saw - a stranger.

I was so shocked, I even glanced over my shoulder to make sure my eyes weren't playing a trick on me. I wrinkled my nose and pouted my lip, because the Kristi I'd known my entire life was gone, and I wasn't ready for her to leave.

Susie came up behind me and placed her hands on my shoulder. I looked at her reflection, and then my own. I looked like *her*. "Was this on purpose?" I thought.

"You look so beautiful Kristi!" she says to me. All I could reply was, "Yeah...right."

On the drive back to my house, I starting working on making the best of it. "O.K.," I thought, "my hair is different. But, maybe it's better!" Dad would surely love it, and boy, would my brothers be surprised.

When we got home, I worked to be mentally ready to be presented to 'the guys'. Slowly I walked up to the house, shuffling my feet, kicking the rocks. I ran my fingers through my hair, gently pressing around the tight curls.

"Ugh," I thought. "It's so SHORT!"

But I kept repeating to myself what Mom had said about fresh starts, and instead of showing everyone how much I hated my hair, I put my chin up, bolted through the door and ran into the house. Without even stopping to see my dad, I ran past the kitchen and barged in to surprise my brothers.

"1-2-3....Taaaa Daaaaa!" I shouted, twirling circles around the room with all the confidence I could muster. They just looked at each other, put their hands over their mouths, and tried unsuccessfully to muffle their laughter. After a few seconds, they broke out in song.

"THE SUN WILL COME OUT - TOMORROW, TOMORROW" they sang, mocking me, and with contemptuous, sarcastic fervor, my jarringly short, curly new do.

"You look like a boy!" Jason shouted. That I could live with. It was the Little Orphan Annie reference that really got to me. I stuck out my tongue and left the room.

"What do they know?" I asked myself. But inside, the answer quickly followed, *"Everything."*

It wasn't long before school started, and I was still embarrassed about my 'Annie' hair. Unlike my bumps and my weight, this was something I couldn't hide under a baggy shirt. I actually tried to pull my hair straight. Ouch.

Just before school started, Susie introduced me to Lisa, her friend's daughter who was just a year younger than me. She thought we'd make great pals, I guess. For my part, I hate being forced to do anything, and wasn't exactly open to my new play partner.

Sometimes, though, when you least expect it, lightning strikes. Lisa and I struck up a friendship that has lasted for over twenty years.

Dressing for the first day of school was easy this year. Instead of sorting through holey jeans and mismatched tops, I was able to prepare the perfect outfit, and walked into Mrs. Adams class with my head held high. I didn't mind being the new kid this year because, for all I knew, everyone was new.

I clenched my new backpack tight around my shoulders, and went up to my new teacher. She was busy talking with other kids who she obviously knew from the year before. When I squeezed myself in and said hello to her, she smiled one of those fakey smiles, and I could tell she was already overwhelmed.

I just raised my eyebrows at her and went to find my seat. It had a name tag on the desk with my name misspelled, but I didn't care. I took my pen and scribbled out the extra letter and put my brand new school supplies inside my desk.

In school, I became known as the 'funny one' - always cracking jokes at myself, trying to let the other kids know that I was okay with being different. But inside, all I wanted was to be just like them: *normal*.

Even though I fought it, I guess Susie putting me into Girl Scouts counts as 'normal', and I really enjoyed my time with the other girls. We went on camping trips, I earned my share of badges, and that spring, I was one of the top cookie sellers in my troop. Susie, either out of a desire to be a good stepmother, or a desire to eat a ton of cookies, helped with this by being the one who purchased half of the orders.

I was short and chubby, while my classmates looked, well, just *better*. At least better than me. Mrs. Adams sat me next to a boy (of course) who immediately began making fun of me. "Ewww!" he'd say whenever my elbow slid past the halfway marker on our desks. Clever boy.

As much as I tried to study and learn, facts and figures just wouldn't stick. I pretended to understand things when they were taught, but as soon as test time came I would panic, because I couldn't remember any of the material.

I was very disorganized and was always losing things. My dad would say "You're just like your brother Mike." I hated that. I loved Mike, but knew he was different from other kids.

Since I always felt like Dad thought Mike wasn't good enough, I wondered - was I not good enough, either? The complexities of parenthood make much more sense to me now, as a mom to six, than they did then. But in that moment of time, I was hurt, regardless of my father's actual motivations and feelings.

Fifth grade was a lot more challenging than fourth, and I wasn't always on the same page as the rest of the class. A particularly embarrassing moment happened when Mrs. Adams brought me up to the front of the class and asked me to find Greenland on the large world map she had pulled down in front of the chalkboard. I searched for about thirty seconds with no luck. She told me to try again. A minute went by, and still no Greenland. The recess bell rang just in time. "Saved!" I thought.

She stopped everyone in their tracks, announcing that until I found Greenland, no one would be headed outside.

"Come on Kristi – it's right there!" The kids were pointing, but still, no luck. Eventually, I did find it, and was pretty annoyed at Mrs. Adams when I did. How was I to know it was, on the map at least, WHITE? I was looking for something GREEN. Sheesh.

Midway through first semester, curiosity got the best of me (big surprise) when I was given a sealed envelope marked "To the parents of Kristianne Hill" to take home to my parents. I carefully opened it in hopes of being able to covertly reseal it. My teacher had a lot to say about me. Apparently, she felt I had trouble remembering what we'd learn from day to day, and in her note to the parents, she indicated I was "lazy and inattentive."

Little did she realize, the more I tried to pay attention, the harder it became. I had even resorted to cheating on some of the weekly tests, just to prove that I was 'smart'. The girl I sat next to had no idea that her answers became mine. I didn't know what else to do. Studying did no good for me. Why couldn't I just be like the others? Why were things so easy for them, but so hard for me?

My attitude slowly transformed from "I can do anything!" to "I really don't care". I was put in weekly counseling to talk about why I was not applying myself. I would get dropped off, then picked up an hour later. The counselor smelled like perfume and mothballs, and, in my eyes, was not the nicest person in the world.

"Why do you think you are here, Kristi?" she asked.

"I don't know. Why AM I here?" As far as I was concerned, I didn't have the problem. She wanted me to talk about how awful my mom must have treated me, and all my problems in school. I stonewalled, telling her only how much I wanted to see Mom, and that school was going just peachy, thank you.

It seemed like she was trying to create a problem for me. That really bugged me. Sometimes I'd hide in the bushes, pretending to go to my appointments, but really sitting at the nearby picnic table drawing cartoons and writing nonsensical paragraphs so my counseling journal looked used. When the counselor called Susie to ask why we had missed two appointments in a row, I was in big trouble – and loudly told how unappreciative and disrespectful I was for skipping them. Hmmph.

CHAPTER 5
Camp Rainbow

The summer of 1986 proved to be life-changing.

When I heard that I could go with Mike and Jason to Camp Rainbow, I was so excited! They had gone the year before, which meant I had heard how great camp was for 12 long months. I was psyched up for something amazing!

Despite that foreknowledge, at first I didn't understand what the camp was really all about. After the bus ride to the camp grounds, it soon became clear this wasn't your 'typical' camp.

Camp Rainbow was for kids facing obstacles of all kinds, from NF to Cerebral Palsy to Cancer. As I glanced around me, I saw campers walking around with braces on their legs, others who were blind, being led by adult counselors, and even a few who had clear plexiforms on their faces (not that I knew that word yet – they were just odd bumps to me). I remember looking around feeling like I should pretend to limp - or maybe I could grab my brother's elbow and pretend to be blind. After all, Mike and I were pros at that game. Of course, I fit in more than I knew.

Once we were assigned our cabins I raced towards mine, leaving my brothers to head their own way. Everyone was yelling "I get top...I get top!" So I yelled that too, though I admit I wasn't totally sure what it meant. When the doors to the log cabin opened, the musty smell hit me and I saw what they were talking about. At least 10 bunk beds lined the walls of the room, each bed decorated with a gift and a new pillow.

My eyes wide, I raced for a bed. Though I ended up with a bottom bunk, I threw my bags onto the mattress and gratefully grabbed my gift.

"Rainbow Brite is my favorite!" I said as I hugged my new doll. I had never actually before seen or heard of Rainbow Brite, but right then and there, she became my favorite.

Our cabin counselor came in to introduce herself, and told us we were going to be the coolest cabin ever! We practiced a song that would become the theme music we'd sing throughout the week. After a few rounds, a loud bell sounded, signaling us to come to the mess hall. Thank goodness – I was starving.

Everyone was so loud, banging their forks on the table and chanting. I looked around, just waiting for an adult to come stop this. To my surprise it never happened, and everyone just kept having fun. The camp leader came in and – get this - STOOD on the table! My mouth dropped open. He took a bucket and a spoon and banged them together. *CLANG* *CLANG *CLANG* "I have some announcements...."

Everyone laughed and cut him off. All at once they sang, "Anouncements, Anouncements, Annnouu-nnccccceeee-ments! A horrible way to die...a horrible way to die...a horrible way to start the day, a horrible way to die."

"How weird!" I said to the freckled, brown-haired girl sitting next to me.

"Yeah, we do this every time they make announcements," she explained. "My name is Jeanie, I was here last year."

I became good friends with Jeanie. We hung out together, inseparable the entire week, whether we were swimming, playing games, or just walking around talking.

The next few days were loaded with so many activities. We'd wake up at 7 a.m. just to squeeze everything into the day.

One of the coolest parts of the camp were the movie stars who would show up throughout the week. Everyone would run to get pictures with them. Finally, being small and short worked in my favor as I slipped through crowds of kids to reach the front of the group.

I hadn't watched many movies at that point in my life, despite living next to the drive-in theater the year before, but I was aware of big names and faces. Ted McKinley (who I knew from *Revenge of the Nerds*), Judith Light (*Who's the Boss*) Kim Fields (Tootie in *The Facts of Life*), James Brolin (From *Hotel* - which I never watched, but the man was gorgeous and I followed him around like I was a lost puppy...He even showed me the inside of his limo!), Todd Bridges and Danny Cooksey (Willis and the cute redhead kid from *Diff'rent Strokes*, respectively), Tom Hattom (Who hosted the *Popeye Show* in Hollywood), Los Angeles Laker's star Kareem Abdul-Jabbar, Heather Locklear (from *T.J. Hooker*), and my heroine, 'Punky Brewster' herself (Soleil Moon Frye), all had roles in my star-studded summer!

Wednesday was Pajama Day, and I'd had the lucky foresight to bring my full-length, zip-up, baby-blue jammies with rainbow socks, which won me "Best Jammies". As I walked over to get my award I noticed a bunch of kids surrounding a man in a black hat who was showing off some dance moves. It looked cool, so after collecting my prize, I ran over to the crowd. Again I squeezed my way to the front to get a better view, and was amazed to see none other than the King of Pop himself, Michael Jackson.

"Nooo way! Isn't that the 'Billie Jean' guy?"

The kid next to me gave me this weird look, "Duuuuhhhh".

I jumped up and began shouting with the other kids. Michael was picking kids from the crowd and showing them how to do the famous 'moonwalk', but I wasn't waiting for him to pick me. I ran up to him and smiled wide with my half-toothless grin, and batted my sweet green eyes. Sticking out my tiny hand I introduced myself proudly,"Hi, I'm Kristi!"

In his soft voice, he replied "Hi Kristi, I like your pajamas!"

I shook his hand and remember how weird it felt. It was very cold and clammy, but the excitement took over when he asked if I knew how to do the "moonwalk".

So I showed him my best backwards slide. "Not bad" he said, encouragingly, "not bad!"*

*During the writing of this book, my brothers have broken the news to me that it wasn't actually Michael, but a celebrity impersonator. Alas — he was Michael to ME, and that's what matters. Thppt!

When I got back to the cabin, I was so excited to tell Jeanie about what had happened, but she wasn't there. Little did I know what was happening with her during my fleeting moments of fame. Full of blissful ignorance, I went to sleep that night happier than I had ever felt.

Morning came too soon. The sound of the bells calling us to breakfast interrupted sound sleep. I crawled out of bed to get dressed and noticed that Jeanie's bed hadn't been slept in. At the foot of the bed, her daily gift still lay untouched. I asked my counselor where she was, then grabbed her gift and ran out of the cabin, headed straight for the nurse's station.

She'd spent the night receiving her chemotherapy, and was very sick. Her eyes were dark and she wouldn't smile at me. I slipped her gift behind my back and walked over to her. She smiled a little, and tried to peek. I laid the stuffed toy on her lap and told her I missed her. The nurse told me that Jeanie would be done and could leave soon, so I sat and waited until she could.

The day promised to be exciting because it was our camp shaving cream fight! Hundreds of cans of shaving cream were placed in huge buckets, waiting for us to let loose and get as messy as possible. The 'no rules' rule made this the best time ever. After the 'fight', the field looked like Christmas morning, covered in a sheet of foamy white snow. Jeanie and I looked at each other and just laughed as we donned white beards and poofy mustaches.

I barely saw Mike and Jay during the week. This became my time to just be me, to just be able to be a kid. There were no worries here. I wasn't afraid of what people thought about me, or who I was going to make angry. I was having so much fun, I never wanted to go home. This was the perfect place for me. A place where hopes could build, and spirits could be lifted. Where even the sick children never really seemed sick. But just as morning had come too soon, so did reality.

The very last day of camp, Jeanie collapsed in the mess hall. Her food tray fell to the floor, her macaroni splatting against the wall. I got up from my seat and ran over to her. She wouldn't wake up.

I didn't understand what was wrong, just yesterday she was running and playing and having fun. One of the counselors quickly carried Jeanie back to the nurse's station.

That was the last time I had with Jeanie at camp. I only knew she was okay when she left the camp because she left a note for me on my bed. Along with the note was the Polaroid I snapped of her the first night we met. As I looked at her picture, I remembered the few short days we spent together. She was so full of life. Her happiness made ME happy.

When I got home from camp that summer, I wrote to Jeanie. I wanted to know if she was okay, and if she had started school yet. I asked about boys in her class and if she liked any of them. I mentioned a few in mine and how immature they all were and thanked her for being my friend, telling her how much fun I had with her at camp.

A few weeks later, I got a letter in the mail. I ripped open the envelope and began to read. I immediately noticed the nice handwriting and was confused when the letter began, "Dear Kristi, This is Jeanie's mother..."

Jeanie had died just a few weeks after coming home from camp. Her mother wanted me to know, though, that all that Jeanie could talk about was her friend Kristi from camp, and she told me how nice it was that I had sent a letter to her.

At that point in my life, Jeanie was the first person I had ever known to have died. I didn't grasp how sick she really was, and I began to feel guilty for not spending more time with her. I got out my scrapbook from camp and placed Jeanie's picture inside it. She will always be a part of my life.

I knew she was sick, and she knew she was sick, but she didn't let that stop her from living. Her mom said Jeanie had

Leukemia and this camp was her final wish. Amazingly, this had been her final wish the year before too! Her illness was something she had to deal with, but it wasn't going to stop her from doing what she wanted to do.

Even now, when things get really bad for me, I think back and remember Jeanie. Her peaceful and loving spirit, how she made me feel so welcomed, *how she unknowingly inspired me to Thrive.*

CHAPTER 6
Private Eyes and Pool Parties

The ringing phone brought devastating news - Mike had been in a bicycle accident. His blinded right eye led him to mistakenly ride our brother Kyle's Mongoose bike off a loading dock, crashing to a concrete landing four feet below.

It seemed like forever before I was able to see him. He was in critical condition, head wrapped in a pile of bandages, but thankfully, he was still Mikey. The doctors told my dad that the shunt that was placed in Mike's head years before had saved his life. Without it, he would have surely died. Ironic - Neurofibromatosis led both to the accident through the blindness and to his rescue, by way of the shunt.

The crash was horrible, and Mike can't remember much of it. It did leave a permanent and painful mark, however. The fall crushed the delicate structure of his ear bones, rendering his right ear completely deaf.

I held Mike's hand and told him that I couldn't wait for him to come home. It was weeks before he finally left the hospital, and still longer before he was back to his usual hijinks.

Entering sixth grade I was definitely not one of the popular kids, but at least I was going to the same school that I had the year before. I began feeling better about myself, and with newfound confidence, ramped up my class clown act from the previous year to a bona fide smart aleck status.

Mrs. Shook offered the perfect classroom environment for me to get mileage out of my growing sarcastic and rebellious nature. I loved to make fun of her for having our classroom decorated with posters of who she called "Her dream man". She even tried to give us a pop quiz based on her Hollywood crush. Everyone in my classroom laughed when I slammed the quiz on my desk.

"A quiz about Tom Selleck, are you serious!?" I threatened to go to the office and report her. Unfazed, she sent me to the Principal herself. I ended up getting lectured about my lack of respect and sentenced to three days of in-school detention. Boy, was I Magnum P.O.'ed!

While most of the girls were into boys and looking pretty, I was content playing with my Barbie dolls. Lisa and I would play for hours, making up stories and pretending their lives were our own. They were so pretty and perfect, it was easy to slip away into their fantasy world.

I was aware playing with dolls was not what everyone else was doing at my age, but I didn't care. I wasn't into makeup and shopping and all the drama of school relationships. Spending time with Barbie and her friends worked for me.

That Spring, I begged for a end-of-the-school-year bash. I didn't think Susie and my dad would actually say yes! Even when they did, I still knew that only a few people who would actually show up. In a surge of optimism, I gave the whole 6th grade an invite to the party.

On the big day, I was moping around the house, worried I would be partying all by my lonesome. Susie had gone out and bought a ton of food – hot dogs, hamburgers, chips of every kind, and enough pop to quench an army.

"Great," I thought. I just knew no one was going to come. With every tick of the clock, I felt the knot in my stomach tighten. I had invited the most popular kids in school - what was I thinking?

Mercifully, the doorbell rang and a few kids trickled in. Thank goodness – I wouldn't be shut out today! Then a few more. Before I knew it, the backyard was turned into a scene from Animal House, with swimsuits instead of togas. It was the most miraculous event I had ever seen! Even Mrs. Shook showed up, though Mr. Selleck was nowhere in sight.

Just when I thought it couldn't get any better, FOUR of the boys I had crushed on all year showed up! I told my dad to keep his camera on them, whispering, "Especially Carrick, the one with orange shorts and red hair."

Now, a party isn't truly hip unless you play the ultimate party game: Spin the Bottle. We all sat in a circle on the grass and took turns spinning a 2-liter of orange soda. Round and round it went, until the bottle rested, clearly pointing at Ernest, a tall and lanky big-eared boy, who was smart and funny. The best thing about him was he never bothered making fun of me. We got our peer-pressure driven hug out of the way quickly, and I kept praying for the bottle to land on Carrick, who I had 'seriously loved' for over a year. This was no secret to my friends, who were cheering for my opportunity to arrive.

When it finally did happen, I signaled my dad to get his camera ready, but he never saw me. He was too busy flipping burgers for the masses. Our special hug was lost in a plume of ashen, barbecue grill smoke.

That's the *public* version. I'll let the rest of you in on what happened next. Spin the Bottle on the lawn is one thing, but it got really exciting when six of us (including Carrick!) headed up to my bedroom. Fate finally favored my fever, and I was able to plant a great big kiss, *on the cheek,* on my fiery-haired flirtation. Only the cruel reality of a poorly designed closet door prevented us from progressing to Seven Minutes in Heaven. Sigh.

For the first time in years, I actually felt normal. I knew how it felt to like and be liked. For that brief afternoon, I was the one who was popular. I wasn't the clumsy, chubby, smart aleck who was always getting into trouble. That day, I was just Kristi, and I was pretty cool.

The summer went by too fast, and before I knew it, I was preparing for Junior High. Lockers, switching classes, and the tragic end of recess. I was excited and nervous. But I was ready to grow up and make lasting friendships, and enjoy some stability. Well, one can hope, right?

Stability took another hit before school started. We packed up and moved from Thousand Oaks to Simi Valley. It could have been worse, though. Susie used her work address and managed to keep me in the same school district, allowing me to stay with my friends.

In her laudable efforts to mother me, Susie kept a tight rein on me, my activities, and my wardrobe. I would often stash clothes I *really* wanted to wear in my backpack, or layer them under the school-marmy dresses she'd make me wear. For the record, designer school-marmy is *still* school-marmy. Once through the front doors of Redwood Middle School, I'd quickly change in the bathroom to the jeans and t-shirts she thought she'd gotten rid of altogether.

Academically, I flew under the radar in 7th grade, as I had the previous few years. I did struggle to keep up, and during one parent/teacher conference, I was again called "lazy and inattentive." What was the deal with this? Do SoCal teachers get a commission for using this phrase? I wasn't lazy. I was doing everything I could to pay attention. Despite this slight hiccup, I managed a C+ average that year, aimlessly floating along from day to day.

Junior High brought with it the inevitable school dance, my first. It was billed 50's Sock Hop. Susie was a whiz with her sewing machine, and she created two amazing poodle skirts for me and my friend Andrea. I wrapped it in a big box and delivered it to her right before the dance.

We dressed up, took the obligatory 'first school dance' pictures, and headed out. No one had actual dates, but we did have our eyes on a few of the boys who would be there. Me especially. I knew Carrick and Jason would be there. I was hoping some of the magic from my party would continue, and one of them would at least talk to me.

I got better than that! Jason invited me out to the dance floor that night. With Kenny Loggins pumping out the theme to Footloose, and our friends all dancing at a frenetic pace, we ignored them all. He put his hands on my hips, I wrapped my arms around his shoulders, and we danced in slow motion, making the most of the three minutes we had together. I floated through the rest of the night, one of my teenage dreams having finally come true.

CHAPTER 7
Worst Year Ever

Another summer brought with it yet another move, this time for a job change. We were moving south to sunny San Diego. I was heartbroken, forced to say goodbye to my hard-earned friends, and to again pack my stuff.

I worked to make the best of it. The house in San Diego was HUGE, and I was happy to again have my own room. I decorated with pictures of my favorite hunks at the time – Chad Allen, Kirk Cameron, River Phoenix, Jon Bon Jovi, and, on the back of my door, Patrick Swayze, in all his full-size, full-length, *Dirty Dancing* glory.

I missed my friends though, and I was scared about starting a new school. Again.

While seventh grade was, perhaps, my calmest year, the upcoming year would prove the cliché "the calm before the storm" to be an absolute universal truth.

I don't like to kill the suspense, but I have to say I HATED the eighth grade. And when I say I hated it, I don't mean I didn't like it....I mean I DESPISED it with a HATRED that could only be understood by, well, probably every other eighth grader in the world who wasn't good looking, popular, or fabulously wealthy.

It started with losing Mike. He was really unhappy living with us, and asked Dad if he could go back with Mom. Dad had no problem with this arrangement, to my knowledge. But when I asked if I could go back too, he refused. I wasn't trying to be ungrateful, I just missed my mom, but Dad seemed to feel I was better off with him.

Over the summer, I put on about 15 pounds and was beginning to resent all the moving around. The 'new start' thing was getting really old, and I was running out of ideas of who to turn myself into.

It didn't take long before I was hand-picked by a few of the popular boys as a target of torment. "Boom Boom Boom!" was just one of several less than complimentary chants to echo around me as I walked the halls of Spring Valley Middle School.

Walking home from school one afternoon, I noticed a few of these tormentors closing in behind me. "Why don't you look normal?" one asked.

"You're so weird!" another boy said.

Keep in mind, it wasn't NF that was inspiring them to say these things – just my awkward-looking, still slightly pre-pubescent self. I walked faster and faster - but no matter how fast I walked, they easily kept up.

"Come on fatty, we're just having fun!" they yelled.

My face was red and hot, and it was a LONG walk home. I wondered if they were going to follow me the entire way. Suddenly, one boy scooped up a rock and threw it at me, just missing my neck, hitting my backpack instead. The others laughed and began picking up rocks to throw at me.

"Let's see if we can make her run!" Just as the boy said that, one big rock hit me on the back of the head. I turned around and the boys ran away. The throbbing pain I felt as I walked home pulsed through my entire body. I never wanted to go back to school. I was done. I was embarrassed. I was mad. I was hurt – both inside and out.

I never talked to anyone at home about this. My dad's marriage was falling apart, and they always seemed too busy to deal with any of the stuff going on at school. I decided to deal with this on my own
.

The day after the rocks were thrown at me, I wanted to show those boys they had not won. That I was tough! But before I even had the chance to prove anything to those testosterone-filled idiots, the girls decided to throw in their two cents.

While getting dressed for gym class, as I slipped my top over my head, a girl made a comment about my 'dirty back'. (*This is a classic symptom of NF, but none of my doctors had bothered to check it out.*) I was covered with birthmarks, small bumps, and discolorations.

"Ewww, Kristi, You need a bath!" I had never looked at my back before, I mean, who really needs to, right? But I knew I wasn't dirty.

Another girl came up to me, before my shirt had fallen to my hips and poked me, "Yea, and what are all those bumps?"

I just slammed my locker shut, fixed my shirt and walked out of the locker room, my untied shoelaces flying.

I got around the corner, out of sight, and reached my hand up my shirt to feel my back. Tiny bumps all along my spine and my hips startled me. I began to cry, sliding down the wall, putting my head to my knees. Anger was welling up inside me and my heart raced, leaving me breathless.

Working to pull myself together, I tied my shoes and wiped my face. I looked over at the group of girls in my class who were laughing and pointing at me. I wanted to run away. What was happening to me? Why weren't my parents talking to me about it? Why haven't the doctors said anything?

I ignored the calls from my teacher to join the class. I wasn't about to let the other kids see me crying, Lord knows they would tease me for that too. I slipped back in the locker room and just sat on the bench in front of my locker. I was confused and angry. I remembered the day I saw my mom undressing, how I had asked about the bumps on HER.

"Was this the same thing?" I wondered. "Was God cursing ME too?" What had I done to deserve this?

I found my gym teacher in the field watching her class run the dreaded mile.

"You know Kristi, if you don't complete this mile run, you'll get a zero" she said.

"I don't feel good, I need to go to the office." I whined.

I begged her to let me go - but she wouldn't. She just sat me on a bench until class was over. I watched as these thin, pretty girls ran around the track, snickering and looking over at me.

I grew more and more angry and asked for God to just get me through this. "Make them stop!" I whispered, hoping God would hear me, and bring me through this day.

Later, on my long walk home, I felt power and courage well up within me. Yet another boy was apparently hoping to prove his manhood by using a stick to try and trip me. I whipped around, took my glasses off, and looked right into his surprised eyes.

"Why am I was so important to you, that you have to go out of your way to make me feel like crap?" I asked.

He offered no response. My courage growing quickly, I told him to grow up - that one day he would be bald and fat, and would end up being on the receiving end of cruel jokes. I told him to spend his time making fun of somebody else, because I wasn't going to let him affect me anymore. He laughed at me, but I felt much better! I walked home a little taller that day.

I went straight to my room to publicly declare (to the pages of my private journal) that I was no longer going to let these kids affect me the way they had been. I was done with being made fun of! I was determined to show these kids that YES! I was different! And I was okay with it.

The next morning, I got to school early and went straight to the gym. I found my teacher sitting at her desk and told her I was ready to run the mile, if she could track my time. She smiled and we walked out to the field together. Twelve minutes and 45 seconds later, I came huffing and puffing around the baseball diamond. I jogged the last bit of that mile and tagged my teachers hand.

"Good job Kristi!" She smiled at me and jotted down my time.

Even though I knew it was only going to get me a C minus. I was happy I ran. I changed back into my school clothes and headed for the library. Three of the main kids who picked on me were sitting at the front table. I always hated homeroom. It was the first hour of school, and it always got my day off to a horrible start.

But not today. Sitting at our shared tables, I just stared at the three boys who were chatting. I smiled sweetly and raised my eyebrows at one of them, and held my stare.

"Hey!" I said to get their attention. "You really don't bother me anymore, you know that?"

"Whatever..." they just laughed.

"I'm serious, I'm really over you guys." I continued. The class quieted down as the bell rang and I straightened up in my chair. I knew I was going to be okay. I felt better about taking the control and not letting these kids win.

On the walk home that day I was sure I would be in for it. I kept looking behind me, waiting for the boys to show up. But they never did. In fact the rest of the school year those boys left me alone.

The girls in gym class, however, continued their tormenting ways. A testament to the persistence of the female gender, I suppose.

Every jumping jack was commented on, every lap around the track snickered at. One day, after a lap around the field, I tried a trick I had heard about to get me out of running. With my breathing fast and my heart pounding, I bent over and held my breath for as long as I could.

I got dizzy and fell to the ground. I woke up with my entire class hovering over me. One girl kicked me with her foot. "Get up lard ass."

The other girls were laughing at me. "She's so fat, she can't even run a lap."

I slowly got to my feet and another girl walked me to the nurse's office. My plan worked. This 'episode' got me out of gym class the rest of the year. But, even with this victory, eighth grade seemed like an eight month death march.

Jay and Kyle had joined the Army and would be leaving soon for Boot Camp. I begged them to stay, but I knew they had to go. Without them, Mike still with Mom, I felt alone.

When the morning came for Jay and Kyle to leave, I prayed harder than I ever had before for something to happen to keep them home. The U.S. was in the middle of the first invasion of Iraq, and I was terrified of what could happen to them. I cried, and hugged them both. They just told me to be strong and that I would make it through this. *Where was my jump rope when I needed it?*

I was tired of just making it through. Tired of everyone messing up my life. What was I going to do without my brothers? When the car pulled away, my face puffed red, I ran to my room and began angrily throwing my stuff in boxes.

I prayed again, "Lord bring them back!" As I was emptying my bookshelf, into the big box that was on my bed, I looked out my window. The military transport that picked them up had turned around. "THEY'RE BACK!" I shouted. I ran out of my room and out the front door, still crying, but with a huge smile on my face.

Jay got out of the car and headed towards me. "Hey sis, I just forgot something", he said as he patted my head. He walked inside, then walked back out.

"Don't leave me!" I begged, trying again to hold them back. Crushed, I sat on the curb in tears, my mind racing with horrible possibilities.

In the long run, our family was fortunate, and both my brothers returned safely after their military service. For that I am grateful.

But as a teenager, the only thing I had to be grateful for that year was the end of eighth grade. Summer couldn't come soon enough.

CHAPTER 8
A Rolling Cone Gathers No Moss

Dad and I moved out of the house and headed to a town called Poway, California. Over that summer Dad and I worked together to lose a few pounds. It turned out to be some good Daddy/Daughter time, something I desperately wanted.

I began to grow out my hair, but my braces were still in, and I still hadn't rebuilt my self-esteem from the beating it took during the last school year.

I was really scared about starting Poway High and wished I had my brothers to talk to. Surely they would have given me some great advice – or at least, advice...

The first day of school I was determined to go in by myself. Dad dropped me off and I went directly to the office to get my schedule. The school was enormous. Not knowing anyone didn't help either, and I walked around like a lost little puppy between classes. There was so much to remember - which class was which, where each class was, and which books I needed at any given moment.

I met Wendy in typing class and we clicked immediately. We hung out a lot, and she and some of the other girls would organize fantastic sleep overs. We sang makeshift karaoke into the wee hours of the nights, taping our own music videos (thankfully, in a time long before YouTube), and participated in general teenage girl silliness.

I invited the friends I'd made over for my Sweet Sixteen Party. We danced to Billy Idol and stayed up all night. The girls and I sneaked out to toilet paper a house down the street that belonged to a boy we all liked – what a blast. We also made prank calls to other boys in our class, calling them and slamming the phone down when they would answer.

While my social life was working out well, it didn't take long before my academic troubles began to follow me to my new school. I struggled to keep up with classwork and didn't really understand what was happening in my math and reading classes.

I went to a few of my teachers to talk to them about my struggles, and my math and English teachers took time out for me, allowing me to come in at lunch for extra help. I also did extra credit with the work that I did understand. They understood my difficulties, and appreciated me taking the initiative.

But, not all the teachers were so understanding. One told me to toughen up and do the work like everyone else. "Why should YOU be any different than the others?" I wished then that I could blame my not understanding the material on something - anything! "Don't be lazy, just do the work" he scolded.

I swear, if I hear myself described as "lazy" one more time, I am going to scream!

Up to this point in my life, my financial resources had all relied on those around me. Sometimes we were broke, sometimes we had plenty. I realized that if I wanted any kind of life of my own, I needed my own money.

I had watched the new Dairy Queen being built in the local strip mall, and knew from the minute I saw it that I wanted to work there. The day I was scheduled to interview, I was ecstatic, but also distracted and nervous.

Not just for the job, but I was trying to win tickets to a James Taylor concert. I kept calling in to my favorite radio station, working to be the 'lucky 7th caller', even while wondering what my interview would be like. When I finally got through and won my prize, I was really shaky, and the hosts of the show asked me what I was so nervous about. I mentioned the interview, and they told me to call them if I got the job.

The next day, I was hired, and called in to report back to my radio heroes. They remembered me, and cheered me on. They even came in later that week for a Peanut Buster Parfait!

While I learned every aspect of DQ operations, I rapidly became famous for a less technical part of my job: wearing the giant plastic cone costume. I stood out on the street corner for hours encouraging motorists to stop what they were doing and take a break. For an ice cream cone, it was incredibly hot to wear, and smelled like nasty old sweat socks.

One time I got knocked over by some clown walking past me. Laying flat on my back, unable to get up, I just played along. I didn't really have much of a choice. I couldn't get the harness off, and eventually I started rolling across the parking lot. Someone finally saw me and propped me back up. My co-workers, though, were no help at all. "Yeah, we saw you!" they said. "We just wanted to see what was going to happen to you!"

Gee, thanks guys. Most of the time, however, I loved my job, and I was making and saving money in hopes to eventually buy my own car, and my freedom.

Ninth grade was the first time boys started paying attention to me for reasons other than to make fun of me. I dated a couple of different young men, including James, who Wendy had briefly went out with before I did, with her blessing.

James and I weren't together very long, but long enough for me to get my first official kiss.

I also decided to go far outside what I thought was my comfort zone, and scheduled myself into Drama 101. Since everyone in the class got a part, I didn't have to be pretty, or skinny, or even funny – I just needed to prove myself on stage. The better I was, the better my part.

We did several plays that term, and I finally got the lead in a play called " A Raisin in the Sun", which was actually kind of bizarre, seeing as the play was about an African-American family living on the South Side of Chicago in the 1950s!

Learning the accent for 'Mama' was a lot of fun, and I can still call upon my 'down home' voice upon request. My ability to cry on cue also gave me my shot in a one-woman skit where I played a dead person looking down on my family as they watched me flatline in surgery. Uplifting, isn't it?

Ninth grade went well, and I felt I was beginning to get my feet on the ground going into the first few days of my sophomore year.

But Dad suddenly had a career change, and we needed to pack up yet again. I was not happy about having to leave my friends, but what could I do about it? I had worked really hard to fit in and now I needed to start all over again. AGAIN.

This time we headed back to Thousand Oaks to live with my Aunt, until we were able to get settled.

When I realized I was going to be able to connect with old friends from 5th, 6th and 7th grades, I started to lighten up, and even look forward to it.

It wasn't the same though. Everyone had grown up. They were so different than they were just a few years before. I was still short and chubby, but the other girls had seemingly turned into full grown women. While I did connect with a few old friends, we had literally grown too far apart.

I fought to keep up with school work, but constantly felt left behind. I turned in assignments late, or incomplete, and I was failing Spanish. Again, I worked out a plan to do extra work to get a passing grade with my Spanish teacher, and it had become a habit to do as much extra credit as possible to keep things going well in my other classes.

Sometimes I felt I just couldn't keep up with any of the work. "What's wrong with me?" I know now that I suffered from a variety of learning disabilities, including Dyslexia and Attention Deficit Disorder.

Regular headaches certainly didn't help either. I was so busy trying to be normal, to not complain, I didn't realize it was okay for me not to be normal, and that I could have gotten help. Instead, I compensated on my own, as best I could.

I was back to hating school, and couldn't wait for it to be over.

Midway through 10th grade, one of my friends asked me about the upcoming SAT testing, and I had no clue about the concept behind this exam. She was studying and asked me to go with her one Saturday morning. She seemed so stressed out about the test, which really confused me. "It's just a test," I thought. "What's the big deal?"

About a month later, I got an envelope in the mail with the test results. 1420 on math and verbal. Honestly, this meant nothing to me, nor did anyone else say anything about it. I folded the paper and stuck it in a stack with other papers.

Much like my NF, it got buried under the drama of my everyday life. Years later, it was brought to my attention that scores that high could have landed me some scholarship money – that despite my challenges in school, I had it in me to be more than I was being.

I liked living with my Aunt Verna. She loved to entertain, and life there seemed to be one party after another. Her house was warm and inviting, and equipped with a huge swimming pool - everyone always had a great time there.

My Aunt is a very spiritual woman, who loves the Lord. I learned a lot about faith the year we lived with her. My perception of God was not positive – and when it came to NF, it was downright negative.

With my only spiritual grounding being a combination of my mom's blaming Him for all the bad things NF caused, and an inconsistent church life that comes with moving year after year, seeing Aunt Verna be so strong in her faith really piqued my curiosity.

Her house was decorated in crosses and pictures of Jesus. I remember a painting hung in her living room. It was of Jesus coming out of the clouds, holding out His arms. I used to stare at this picture and remember feeling so confused. Could He really be to blame for all of our problems?

I survived the year, and enrolled in summer school for math and Spanish, in an effort to keep myself on track. But, summer would bring with it yet another move. Dad got a job that moved us to Colorado Springs.

After two years living back with Mom, Mike decided he wanted to move with us to Colorado, and Kyle was also heading to the Springs, having returned from his stint in the military with honors. Having two of my three brothers made the transition a little easier, but I was tired of moving, of having to start over one more time.

Just before starting school in Colorado, I headed back to California to spend two weeks with my mom. Even though Mike had been living with her, we had had virtually no contact since I had moved out the summer after fourth grade.

It was so great to see her again. I shadowed her at the daycare center she worked at, helping her teach a preschool class. I loved it – it was the first time I realized how much I loved working with kids. The director thought I had done so well, she offered me a job.

This appeared to me to be a significant opportunity – a chance to break out of my academic torture, to gain independence, and continue to reconnect with Mom. After a few long, late night talks, I decided I would take my General Educational Development test and move in with her.

My only hurdle? Telling Dad, who was briefly back in town on business. We met at Denny's for breakfast. Before I began to talk with my father, I gobbled up a bit of my eggs and pancakes for strength. I then gulped my orange juice and quickly laid out my plan. I was sure I had it all figured out, and he would agree it was a fabulous idea.

The look in his eyes told me he didn't think it was so fabulous. From my perspective at the time, it was a look of a man betrayed, a look of utter disgust. I felt I had disappointed him.

"Why would you want to do this after what happened? How could you do this?" he said, glaring at me from across the table. I tried to reason with my father, but he slammed his napkin down and got up from the table and walked away, leaving his plate of half eaten fried eggs and pancakes. I was heartbroken, and confused.

"How could I do this to HIM?" I thought to myself, tears rolling down my face, "How could HE do this to ME?" For years, move me all over the place, never let me settle down, and then deny me something I had decided I wanted so badly?

Feeling abandoned, I got up from the table. I looked around for my dad, who had paid for breakfast and headed out to the parking lot. I quietly got in the car and we drove back to Mom's. The drive back was awkward and tense. This conversation would never be brought up again, and I dutifully returned to Colorado, leaving the job, my 17 year-old concept of independence, and my mom, behind.

CHAPTER 9
Smarter Than She Looks

After the move, I was angry at the world. Angry at Dad. Angry at Colorado. I didn't want to be there, and I made no effort in making friends. I stayed to myself, and just wanted the year to hurry and get over with. While it was cool having Mike and Kyle there, all I could think about was just growing up and being able to make my own choices.

Despite my efforts at self-isolation, I ended up with a boyfriend. Eric was a shy but good-looking boy, who I couldn't believe was showing interest in me. We dated for most of the year, but I always felt I wasn't good enough for him. He didn't exactly boost my self-esteem, either. At school he barely acknowledged me. When we'd go out, he would always walk ahead of me. I didn't understand how to act with him. Was he just being nice to me, or did he really love me?

For Christmas, Eric surprised me with a puppy. I'd always wanted my own dog, but it had never worked out over the years. I hid in the bathroom, and was called out to find this tiny dog jumping all over the living room. This was truly one of the best gifts I had ever received. I named my new black

Labrador puppy Nicki, and started jumping all around the living room alongside her.

School went fine, and I kept my electives light, focusing on my more difficult subjects. Unexpectedly, my results on a math assessment placed me above grade level. I was sure that this was a mistake. It only took one day in the trigonometry class to know it was far too much. I was quickly plopped back into a regular math class. Whew. Bullet dodged!

On Valentine's Day, Eric took me out. After the movie, we drove around, unsure of what to do next.

"Look in the back seat," he told me. I saw a small white bag. "Look inside."

I fumbled through the bag and saw a small collection of sex toys he had purchased. Yikes! Was THIS what he wanted? We had barely begun kissing and now he is pushing for SEX? With TOYS?

"Take me HOME," I demanded.

I wasn't about to have this be the start of my sex life. Eric drove me home, apologizing and rubbing my hand. He parked in front of my house, and begged me to forgive him. We ended the night with a soft kiss, but I felt cheapened and confused. Why would he think that was okay? We didn't break up over what happened that night, but it did change my opinion of him, and put me more on my guard.

That summer Kyle made plans to buy and build a house. My father began talking about – yes - another move. I would be 18 soon, and told him I was done with moving. Kyle said it would be okay if I rented a room out of his new house. I'd finish school, keep my boyfriend and finally create stability.

But, as the summer moved on, I felt less and less comfortable with the idea of staying in Colorado. Kyle had his own life going on, and Eric and I were not exactly Romeo and Juliet.

Mike would be going with Dad, and I found myself torn. Maybe it was just what I had grown accustomed to, but I changed my mind and decided to move to Utah after all.

Even though it was my decision, I was frustrated. We had to leave a lot of stuff behind – including my green Diamondback bike. If only that truck had had an extra foot!

Despite my intentions at the beginning of the year to avoid building friendships, I was sad to let go of the friends I'd developed after all. I gave my puppy away, and broke the news to Eric. Breaking up with him wasn't as tough as I thought it would be.

"Okay," he said. "I'll miss you." No fighting for me, no tears. John Cusack with a boom box he was not.

Not long after we arrived in Roy, Utah, Dad took me down to the local car lot and bought me my first car (for some reason, I never did save enough working for Dairy Queen to buy my own. Go figure).

I picked out a 1980 poop-brown Chevy Monza. The car was awesome, and it was MINE! Even with tacks holding the inside roof together, and its easy, no-key-necessary starter system, it almost made moving worth it. I loved that car!

Truthfully, it did make my transition a little easier, and my respect for my dad increased. He saw what having some freedom meant to me, which meant he was starting to see ME, and what I needed.

I was determined to make him proud, so without hesitation I registered myself right away at Roy High School.

The guidance counselor looked at my school records and told me I was just a few credits away from having all I needed to graduate, but handed me a full schedule of classes anyway. I walked out, not excited about the 7 courses I saw on the paper, including a class called Seminary. What was THAT about? I later discovered it was a religion class held at the nearby Church of Latter-Day Saints, and all the LDS students took it each term. One problem: I was not LDS. Epic fail, RHS.

Halfway to my car, I stopped, turned around and walked back into the school with new resolve. I stopped my counselor, just as she was leaving.

"Is it really necessary for me to have ALL these classes? I mean, I only need 3 credits to graduate. Can't I do, like, work study or something?" I asked.

"If that's what you want." she huffed, rolling her eyes.

I smiled. "Yep, sign me up!"

In hindsight, I wonder what would have happened had this counselor taken the time to explain to me her reasoning behind the class schedule, to enlighten me as to my academic potential. She had access to my grades, my challenges, my test scores, but didn't bother to guide OR counsel me.

Looking back, no one in my life had taken enough notice of what I was capable of. They were too busy with medical issues and job issues and relationship issues - just too busy with life. And I was too busy surviving year to year to find out for myself - a mistake I would continue to make for far too many years.

With just a few taps on the computer, I was enrolled in an evening art class, and I could earn the remaining two credits by working. Next stop? Get a job. I immediately drove down the street to the local Dairy Queen.

"I can do this!" I said to myself. Why not? I'd done it before. I parked, walked in, and confidently asked for the manager. He asked about my experience and I told him about my DQ days back in San Diego. I was hired on the spot and started work the next day. Lucky for me, they didn't have an ice cream cone mascot suit to be worn!

My excitement was quickly dulled by my dad's lack of enthusiasm. I knew he was just afraid that I was missing out by not attending regular school my Senior year. He didn't seem to understand that I didn't want to start new, to be the new kid - AGAIN. It wasn't pleasant, but I stood up for what I thought was best, and he eventually let me make my own choice.

Working at DQ was easy and fun - and living in Utah wasn't as bad I imagined. I made several friends at work, and even became comfortable enough to revert back to my younger, more outgoing persona of Krazy Kristi!

A few girlfriends from work invited me over for a slumber party, and the night started getting rowdy. Truth or Dare turned into Dare Krazy Kristi – because she'd do anything!

Finally, they dared me to run around the block. In the cold. Without my top. I figured, hey, why not? It was late, it was dark, who was there to see? Nobody. At least until my last few yards back to the house, when my friend's brother showed up. Sheesh! The legend of Krazy Kristi grew exponentially that night.

My art class lasted for six weeks, and I easily earned the necessary work study credits in a few short months. After being held back in second grade, after struggling year after year, I was actually going to graduate EARLY!

I didn't attend any courses during the Spring, but I did walk the stage with my graduating class. I wanted to give my Dad the full cap and gown experience – and it was pretty cool having people whispering "Who the heck is she?" as I accepted my diploma.

I received my summary transcript, a long document listing all four high schools. I ended up with a 3.85 GPA. Just like the SAT scores, this meant nothing to me, and nobody chose to enlighten me. I was just happy to be done with school – FOREVER!

CHAPTER 10
Two Kids and the Christmas Tree

By the time my 19th birthday came, my life had calmed down. Dare I say I felt stable?

I had left Dairy Queen for a higher-paying opportunity with Wal-Mart, working as a cashier and occasionally manning the snack bar.

I parted ways with my trusty Monza, trading up for a White Honda CRX. This car was even cooler than my first, and I felt 'grown up' when I qualified for a loan all by myself, my monthly payment only $82. Well worth it – I loved cruising around town in my new baby.

In 1993, I met Troy. He worked at Wal-Mart too, and we hit it off right away. I liked him a lot - he was tall and strong and protective of me. He wore a black cowboy hat and made me mix tapes of his favorite songs. This was the first time I'd ever had this kind of relationship; it felt really nice.

It wasn't too long before he proposed, right in front of his parents, in the living room of their house. The ring sparkled and I slipped it on my finger. Teary-eyed, I reached up to hug him, and said "Yes."

We didn't get married right away, partly because my father wasn't on board. To my surprise, he actually suggested we move in together first. Perhaps he hoped that would snap me to my senses.

I was a bit confused, but I was engaged, and desperately wanted my own life. Troy and I moved in together, and before long, I discovered I was pregnant. We were both excited and scared about the prospect of a baby.

Unfortunately, I miscarried very early on. It was heartbreaking, and neither Troy or I were well-equipped to handle it.

I didn't tell very many people about that pregnancy, both because it ended before I could emotionally digest that I was ever pregnant, and because living together with Troy led to a tremendous guilt within both of us.

We had told our landlady we were married, and we were attending a church where it was also assumed we were married. Even at 19, I knew this was not the way I wanted to start my family life.

We decided to go ahead with wedding plans, but I was scared to tell Dad that I didn't want a big wedding. I just wanted to get it over with and make it legal. One Saturday, Troy and I eloped in his parent's backyard.

When the minister asked "Who gives this woman in holy matrimony?" there was only uncomfortable silence. After a few seconds, Troy's father piped up. "I guess I do." At that moment I regretted my choice. I wanted the white gown. I wanted my dad to walk me down the aisle and give me away. I wanted it to be celebrated and joyful.

The secret of being married was worse to carry around than the secret that I wasn't married. Inside, I knew it was wrong to do, and felt terrible for going through with it. I hid my ring so no one would see it, but I was dying inside.

One day in front of my apartment, I told my father about our secret wedding. The look on his face was the same as if I had told him someone died. I had deeply hurt him. He drove away, leaving me sitting on the curb. I cried and felt hopelessly alone.

As I sat with my thoughts, I knew my dad only wanted what any father wants for his daughter. The dream man who will lead and take care of his baby, the fairy tale wedding, where he walks his daughter down the aisle and gives her away, gently kissing her cheek as he hands her off. I had ruined that for him. I had ruined it for me.

Even though I understood that, all I really wanted at that moment, as any daughter wants from her father, was a comforting hug. For him to tell me everything was going to be okay, whether he thought so or not.

I changed jobs often those first years of marriage, never sure of what I wanted to do in life. I had always dreamed of growing up, getting married, and having kids playing in the front yard of my house surrounded by a white picket fence, with a green minivan parked in the driveway.

Instead, I was working in the Albertson's grocery store bakery.

We weren't really planning on having kids right away, especially after our experience before we married. I was taking birth control pills, but discovered too late that the antibiotics I had taken for strep throat could nullify their effectiveness.

I took a home pregnancy test on Mother's Day of 1995. This news made me surprisingly happy. More than anything, I felt being a mother was what I was meant to be, the one role I could have control over. I worked through four months of my pregnancy, and Troy and I moved to another apartment.

Once I had moved beyond the danger zone, I realized I loved being pregnant. The movement in my belly, the feeling of life growing inside of me, the excuse to eat all the soft serve vanilla ice cream I wanted.

My Obstetrician check-ups were consistently normal, and NF was never mentioned. I had begun to notice more bumps were showing, especially on my back and tummy, but the doctors never brought it up, so I figured I was okay. If they felt there was something wrong, surely they would have taken the time to tell me.

My delivery date was near Christmas, and Dad had bought a 1995 Baby's First Christmas Ornament for his soon to be granddaughter. In her first act of utter defiance, baby waited more than a week. Bailey's 'Papa' was forced to buy a 1996 version, instead. We still hang both on the tree every year.

I was in labor for 19 hours, and gave birth to my beautiful 7 pound 11 ounce baby girl. We brought her home, and I started adjusting to being a mother. I wanted to give Bailey everything.

She and I spent every minute of the day together. As a newborn, she showed no trace of NF, and, as I had been taught to do by my own history, I allowed NF to become a forgotten factor.

A few weeks after Bailey was born, my mother called to tell me she was moving to Utah! She wanted to be closer to me and my growing family. I was shocked, but very happy. I so badly wanted to reconnect with her. She moved into an apartment just 15 minutes away.

I worked hard to create the family I had always wanted, to foster hope and stability. It wasn't always easy. Finances tightened, and as a young couple, Troy and I didn't always work together well.

A year after Bailey was born, I found out I was pregnant again. I prayed that God would give us a boy, thinking that a son might help bring us closer together, and give my husband another reason to connect with me.

I gave birth to our son in early October, 1997, and I had my 'perfect' family. Braden was placed on my belly, with his umbilical still attached. It was the most miraculous feeling I have ever experienced.

The warm, wet body, of this new life now released from my own was clinging to me, and I could feel his heart beating next to mine.

He was absolutely perfect. I examined every bit of his 21 inch body. All 10 toes, 10 fingers, brown hair - with a little cowlick right in front. He had the bluest eyes I have ever seen.

My perfect moment was soon interrupted when my baby boy was whisked away to be cleaned and checked out by the nurses. His Apgar scores were strong at first, then steadily declined. The nurses called for help, then the respiratory team came racing in – and racing out.

The room fell silent, as they finished cleaning up the birth scene and assembling the bed. Troy was forced to decide whether to be at our baby's side, or mine.

I soon found myself alone. I looked out the window, it was barely 5 o'clock in the morning and I could see the sun just touching the tips of the Utah mountains. I was exhausted from 21 hours of labor, and found myself drifting into a deep and dreamless sleep. I remember feeling so peaceful and warm.

It didn't last long.

I was jolted awake by Troy's hand on my arm. He was sobbing. He told me that I needed to come see our son. The wheelchair was waiting next to the bed. When we got to the NICU, I was confused. My son was so big and healthy. He was a HUGE baby! How can he possibly be in the NICU? This was a place for tiny preemies, not the beautiful big-headed baby boy I had birthed just hours before!

Yet, there he was. My handsome prince. Tubes were everywhere. One for breathing and many coming out of his umbilical stump. His pediatrician came over to me, to fill me in on what was happening.

"He's very sick." he said. I thought he was mistaken....He must have the wrong baby! Then he said something that would change my life forever. "There's not much hope, I'm sorry."

Troy fell down next to me and hugged me. We both just cried and cried. Then I looked up at my baby. I saw his feet moving and his little hands opening and clenching. All I saw in that little Isolette was hope, and it was pouring out of my son! I wasn't going to let some doctor tell me that there was no hope. How dare he?

Yes, our little big guy was quite sick. Turns out he was born six weeks early due to a miscalculation by my OB. His size had thrown off the calculations, and sadly, we actually sped up the delivery date. It was strange seeing this behemoth baby among many tiny, fragile ones.

Braden had a neighbor in the ICU, a beautiful baby girl, born at 25 weeks gestation. She was barely two pounds. She and my son had very similar breathing problems. I visited with her mother one day. We both sat and held our newborns tight, and our hope even tighter.

Braden spent two very long weeks in the NICU. He was released just before Halloween (no doubt he was determined to go trick or treating!). Before we left, his doctor came to give him a final look over, "he's perfect", he told me. I just smiled and said a silent prayer of thanks.

Two years later, I bumped into the mother I had met at the NICU. I didn't see a child with her, and I was afraid to ask. She recognized me, too, and asked how I was. Braden was pulling at me and whining about an ice cream cone. Just as I was about to answer, a tiny little girl came running up to her mommy shrieking with joy. "This is my daughter, Hope." she announced. Hope was absolutely beautiful.

Over the next few months, life changed significantly. We moved into a bigger apartment and I took on two jobs to augment Troy's income. Braden continued to grow stronger, and with all the other issues surrounding his birth, NF didn't come up with him any more than it had with Bailey.

My brother Mike had been living with Dad, and his appendix abruptly ruptured, causing a seizure. I had come by the house just as his attack was happening, and followed as an ambulance rushed him to the hospital.

An infection was beginning to rage through his body, resulting in a new shunt being installed. Dad ended up deciding Mike needed more professional care, and decided a nursing home was the best place for him.

It tore me up to see my big brother there. My childhood partner in crime seemed so unhappy. Against my dad's better judgment, I signed Mike out of the nursing home and brought him into ours.

There was already distance growing between my husband and me, and bringing Mike into the mix didn't make life much easier. Despite a full house, I felt very alone.

I had done everything I knew to do to make things work, but ultimately chose to end our marriage after almost 5 years. There was no fighting, it was almost as if we both just knew it was over. He moved out just weeks before Christmas.

I was working so much to keep our bills at bay, I didn't realize that I didn't even have a Christmas tree. Now, I'm no Martha Stewart, but I do have an addiction to holiday decoration – and usually begin a good month before the actual holiday. I couldn't believe I had forgotten all about a tree.

A few days before Christmas I headed to the store to see what was left. I found the most beautiful tree I had ever seen - and it was on CLEARANCE! I strung up the lights and the few ornaments that I had onto the tree. The next morning the kids helped string Fruit Loops and gave our tree some healthy, vitamin fortified color.

Troy came over Christmas Eve and stayed the night on the couch. The next day was uncomfortable, but I just kept thinking about Bailey and Braden, and making this the best possible Christmas for them. If they were happy, so was I. During the last few months of my marriage, both Bailey and Braden began showing signs of NF. The cafe au laits spots were picked up at well visits and noted in their charts. Still, I was told not to worry, that the cafe au laits were "no big deal."

Bailey was developing normally, and while Braden fell behind in almost every milestone, it was explained away by his prematurity. Surely he would catch up, he just needed time.

The stress and exhaustion was beginning to affect my health. I had been having more severe headaches than usual. With Mom close by, I was beginning to notice the similarities, both physically and in behavior, between us.

One night after a shower I noticed a tumor on my neck. I pinched and pulled on this growth, then opened my towel to look at my body in the mirror. Tiny bumps I had never before seen, or just never wanted to see, were now very obvious.

I opened the medicine cabinet and took out a razor blade. I washed it clean with soap and water and tilted my head. With one hand I grabbed the tumor, and took the razor blade in my other hand.

Desperate, I sliced through the tumor to remove it from my flesh. I didn't care about the physical pain it caused me, for its mental pain was far worse. Little did I know back then, that this was only one of thousands that would eventually appear all over my body.

The warning signs of NF's invasion of my body were everywhere. But not only was I conditioned to ignore them, I was too scared to acknowledge them. I was determined to keep going.

I added babysitting on top of my two jobs and asked Mom if she'd be willing to move in with me.

She agreed and with her and Mike in the house, I had essentially recreated what I had back when I was young – plus two great little kids.

I admit, I never thought things would be like this. Never thought I'd end up a single mom, struggling to make it. Even so, the struggle was making me stronger everyday.

CHAPTER 11
Striking it Rich with Six

While I wasn't looking for another relationship right away, it didn't take long before one came my way.

I went into 1999 thinking I just wanted to enjoy finding out who I was, and take the time to focus on my kids. I didn't want to bring a guy into the picture, whether it be mine, or Bailey and Braden's. Besides, I thought, who would want me?

Krazy Kristi got the better of me one night, though, and I put an ad out on Yahoo! Personals. I cropped a picture of me in my favorite sweater, put a few details out, and sent it off to whoever might run across it on the web. I figured I might get a date or two off of it, and hey, nothing was wrong with a free dinner or movie, right?

The next morning, my inbox was overflowing with nearly 400 responses! Unbelieveable! What was even more unbelievable was what these people were asking for. One night stands, threesomes, swingers, affairs – and that's just what I can print! Only three responses seemed to come from normal, upstanding citizens.

One of them was a guy named Rich. I replied to him, and we ended up speaking over AOL's Instant Messenger for a day, but neither one of us were interested in hiding behind our computers.

Rich even told me that for all I knew, he was a 3000 pound gorilla, so we ought to get together just to make sure. I replied, telling him for all HE knew I was a 3000 pound gorilla, and dared him to meet me anyway!

We did address some important issues online before we met though. He knew I had two kids, I knew he had one from a college relationship years before. He knew I lived with my mom and brother, and my brother had some challenges. I knew about his own birth defect, which resulted in him having a noticeable limp.

NF didn't come up. In fact, for the most part, NF wouldn't come up at all for far too long.

Two days after sending out that crazy personal ad, I was meeting Rich at Denny's late on a Saturday night – late so that he could make the half hour drive north, and late so I could get the kids down to sleep before I left to meet him. I saw him sitting in his car when I drove up, and when he got out, I tried to hide a smile.

Frankly, he looked better than I expected. I even told him how cute I thought he was, and afterward thought, "did I really say that out loud?"

We sat and talked for almost two hours over a couple of hot chocolates. I was shy, and he seemed so confident. I had my hair up, and he actually asked me to put it down. I couldn't believe he could be that forward, but I went ahead and let my long hair drop around my face. He smiled, and told me I had the most beautiful eyes he'd ever seen.

I insisted on paying that night – it was my own little way of saying I was in control. But, I also gave him a big hug before he left. It was the first time I felt safe in a long while, even if it was only for a few seconds.

The next 11 months were a bit of a whirlwind. Rich and I got serious quickly, and it scared me. I wasn't ready for it all, and during the summer, we actually split up. Rich was persistent though, and our 'break' only lasted a couple weeks before I realized he wasn't going away, no matter how hard I pushed.

After that, we spent a lot of our time together having long conversations geared toward the future. From parenting to money management to family life to religion – nothing was off limits. Rich had just come out of a marriage himself, and said he wanted to put everything on the table. We agreed on just about everything, though his lack of appreciation for Garth Brooks was almost a deal breaker.

The biggest factor in our relationship, beyond ourselves of course, was Bailey and Braden. They took to Rich quickly, and he was more than willing to tackle the challenges of two young kids. He loved to play and roughhouse with them around the house, and wasn't afraid to change a diaper. Having more kids was a desire we both shared, and certainly one that would be quickly fulfilled.

NF wasn't an issue during our courtship. Rich didn't seem to mind my tumors. In fact, he acted like he didn't even notice them. I loved him for that, but inside, thought he was just being nice. I was still very self-conscious about my body. What did he possibly see in me?

In October, he proposed to me in a Park City restaurant, going down on one knee in front of everyone there. I was happy to accept, and couldn't wait to start planning my wedding.

I decided this time, I was going to do it right – church, dress, and most importantly, Dad walking me down the aisle.

December 11, 1999, Bailey, Braden, Rich and I were presented as a family to the small group of friends and relatives who had gathered to witness. I never could have imagined this moment just a year before. I felt closer to my dream life than ever – we were moving into a condo, Rich had a steady job, and stability was again within my grasp.

Dad put on a wedding reception at his house, and kept the kids overnight to let Rich and I have a quick, 24 hour honeymoon. In another few weeks, we realized our brief escape was more productive than we expected, and we were now expecting! Life was not about to slow down, and our daughter Riley was born nine months later.

The next seven years were relatively NF free. While I saw more and more bumps appearing, I didn't say much about it. As long as it wasn't affecting day to day life, I didn't see reason to worry.

Rachel came along in 2002, and had a few of the earmarks of NF, but the doctors weren't concerned, so neither were we. The rest of life was keeping us too busy to worry about it anyway.

In April of 2004, Rich sent me and the kids to Spokane, Washington, where Rich's sister and mother lived. We stayed at his mom's house while he focused on getting the condo sold and looking for a job. He had been laid off from a sales position two months earlier.

We were toying with the thought of moving, feeling a change of pace would do us all some good. The two bedroom condo we were in was shrinking fast, with four kids sharing one bedroom. Things got so desperate we even moved *our* bed into the living room for awhile. NOT a good solution.

In mid-May, I found out I was pregnant with baby number five. We honestly hadn't been planning on another quite yet. I guess when Rich sent me off to Washington, he sent me with a little something extra!

Job hunting wasn't going well, but a deal on the condo was being done, so we decided to take the next big step – move to Washington.

My family wasn't thrilled with me moving the grandchildren 14 hours north, but it was time for me, and all of us, to cut some apron strings. We would still have Rich's family as a support system in Spokane.

June through November, we all lived with Rich's mom. In September, he went to work with an ad agency, and by Thanksgiving, we'd found a duplex to move into. I love my mother-in-law, but I wasn't about to give birth to a new baby in her home.

A few days before Christmas, Riker Jeffrey arrived. Rich is a huge Star Trek fan, and it was all I could do to keep our son from being named James Kirk or Sulu Tiberius! The name fits my boy though – and I couldn't imagine him with any other.

2005 seemed to go by quickly. Neurofibromatosis still wasn't a real issue, at least that we were aware of – but looking back, we should have been. Braden was having major setbacks in school, and it was clear he wasn't mentally maturing as fast as his peers. While a prime red flag as an NF symptom, instead we, and the doctors, chalked it up to his struggles as a preemie.

Rachel had been developing a bit slowly as well, but not at nearly the reduced rate of her older brother. A late walker and talker, her delays were attributed to her small size, and rationalized by Rich and I as her just having a different, less outgoing personality.

Turns out, we were wrong on both counts. Shyness is not one of Rachel's character traits in the least! But at 2-3 years old, we had little reason for concern. Younger brother Riker showed no signs of NF. I knew he could still show signs later on, but it was a worry I left buried under the challenges of daily life with five children.

In January of 2006, an all-new challenge popped up. Rich found himself unable to put weight on his left ankle. He had just hired on at a local magazine, and was suddenly stuck on crutches. He was sure the pain would subside, as he'd had bad days before. The days stretched into weeks, and I finally convinced him to see a doctor. Rich never walked on his left ankle again.

The doctors laid out three options: surgery, that, if it worked at all, wouldn't last more than a year; a full-length leg brace, significantly altering his mobility; or an amputation.

Watching him go through the struggle of making that decision was one of the hardest times of my life. While we made the choice together, how could I truly have any real say over whether or not he should voluntarily cut off his leg?

In April, he went through with the surgery – an upgrade, he called it. By June, he was learning to walk again, and in July he was, for the most part, fully mobile.

Near the end of August, Rich and I had an amputation of another kind on our minds. With five kids and not much money coming in, I felt it made sense to stop the babymaking machine. Specifically, HIS. Ladies, I know you're with me on this one. Guys are big babies about this, even though its so much easier for them to go through a 'snip-snip' procedure than us.

After some convincing, we scheduled the appointment. I promised Rich royal treatment for the next few days, and dropped him off. I was proud of him for making this happen, and I was ready to take the worry of another child off my uterus. When I returned to pick him up -- all hell broke loose.

Rich hadn't done it. He was sitting on the table as I walked in, and when he told me, I flipped. I looked at the doctors and shouted "Where's the knife? I'll do it myself!" I couldn't believe it.

As we headed home he was spouting off his excuses about how he 'wasn't ready', and 'what if you died and I need to remarry so the kids have a mom', and how he felt there was another baby waiting for us. Horsepuckey! Men – can't live with 'em, can't kill 'em.

Sure enough, by September, I was pregnant again. My fault for not staying angry at him long enough, I suppose. I was under a tremendous amount of stress. Our finances were a mess. The people around me couldn't believe I was pregnant again. The ultrasound said otherwise.

There my baby was, its strumming heartbeat filling the room. The moment was filled with calm fear. I didn't know how I was going to handle this, I just knew I would. I had no choice.

Late November proved to be a turning point. I miscarried. It was my fourth miscarriage over the years, but the first whose heartbeat I had heard. It was over Thanksgiving, and I felt I had little to be thankful for. I was heartbroken.

My family and friends thought this would be the final straw, but in fact, I gained strength from the loss. Suddenly, I knew Rich was right – there WAS another baby out there for us. I couldn't bear the thought of leaving a lost soul waiting to join our family.

I told my sister-in-law not to be surprised if she got a call, soon, that I was pregnant again. She looked at me first in shock, then in resignation. Two months later, she got that call, and baby number six was on her way.

While I was happy to again be expecting, home life was still a major challenge. Rich struggled to find steady employment that paid enough to be worth working. In July, he was offered a job that would take him out of town, and keep him out of town, for months at a time. The potential financial return seemed worth it. Still, we struggled with the decision to send him off, leaving me with five kids and one on the way.

He took the job, but it took less than a week for him to turn around and fly back to us. The job wasn't what he expected, and he couldn't handle being away. I was angry that yet another job hadn't panned out, but was also glad to have my husband back. While I was prepared to handle the family and the baby on my own while he worked, inside, I knew he had made the right choice.

Frustrated, and feeling like failures, we returned to Utah. This time we moved in with MY mom, and the next few months proved to be the most stressful of my life.

CHAPTER 12
From Brooklyn to Braden:
The Birthpains of Thriving

One of the first things on my mind when we returned to Utah, of course, was getting an OB/GYN. I tracked down the Obstetrician who had delivered Riley and Rachel, and was relieved that she was more than willing to take me on as a patient again. With less than a month to go, my fear of delivering in an emergency room was finally gone.

I liked my OB. She had always been kind, and had done a wonderful job handling the challenges of my earlier pregnancies. She put in a cervical cerclage to keep me from delivering Riley early, and quickly handled Rachel's early respiratory distress, just minutes after birth. While I had to drive a half-hour to get to her office, I was still happy to have rediscovered a doctor I could count on.

I arrived for my first appointment ready for a thorough exam. I knew she would want to make sure everything was addressed at this late date. Running the Doppler over my 38 week pregnant belly, a puzzled look took over her face. "This looks like Neurofibromatosis," she said, clearly surprised.

I closed my eyes, not wanting to hear that word. I was trapped in silver stirrups, nowhere to run, no covers under which to hide. Didn't she know? Didn't she notice the first two times? Why didn't she see the bumps before - had I gotten worse?

"Well, it's too late to do anything about this now - you're 38 weeks pregnant."

"Too late to do anything? What exactly should I have done?" I asked myself. I knew it would useless to protest. Instead, I just closed my eyes, took a deep breath and told her about my five happy and healthy children at home, and that I expected no different an outcome from this pregnancy.

I could tell she wasn't buying it, and she looked at me with a combination of pity, anger, and judgment. Or maybe she just looked at me, and I saw my own face, my own fears, my own guilt, judging me for hiding for so long.

After I left the doctors office, a crushing realization hit me with such force I could barely drive. I was shaking and crying – I had left NF in my closet for 33 years.

As a child, it was put there by others, but as an adult, I had done nothing to bring it out from its hiding place. I had felt justified. Excused. If nobody could see my NF, my husband, my kids, even my doctors, then maybe I didn't really have it.

That part of me died by the time I pulled into my mom's driveway. In its place, just as my baby had grown in the grief of my miscarriage, a new perspective, a new passion, *a new Kristi*, found life.

I knew I had to accept my reality, even through my fear. Now was the time to do it. No more running, no more hiding. I had brought real people into this world, and they needed a voice.

My voice. Three of them, Bailey, Braden and Rachel had the earmarks for NF (cafe au laits, freckling under the arms and around the neck) but I hadn't taken them in to be officially diagnosed by a geneticist.

After Brooklyn was born, I examined her immediately. With my other children, I knew birthmarks didn't show up until a few weeks after their birth. So, each day I would get my newborn daughter undressed and scan every inch of her tiny, perfect being.

We moved out of Mom's house two months later, down to Provo, Utah. Rich had finally landed a job with the local paper, and for awhile it seemed like life was heading in a positive direction.

But NF could no longer be ignored, if was no longer just MY personal problem. I scheduled all six kids to be examined. The final verdict? Riley, Riker, and Brooklyn were clear of Neurofibromatosis, while Bailey, Braden, and Rachel all showed positive for my family's personal curse.

In truth, I wasn't surprised. Puzzle pieces fell into place. Bailey and Braden both struggled academically. Braden's behavior issues had intensified as he grew older. Rachel? Sadly, she was soon to be the first to feel the impact of NF.

During her initial examination, the doctor noticed Rachel's eyes crossing. While this can be considered normal in children at that age, and easily corrected, her NF diagnosis prompted the doctor to schedule an MRI. They didn't find as much as they expected. The usual UBO's (Unidentified Bright Objects) were present, and her ventricles were underdeveloped. No course of action was recommended, other than yearly MRI's.

By November, 2008, we found ourselves in a position to move yet again. This time, back to Washington. Our year in Utah had not been what we'd hoped. Connecting with family was difficult with the two hour distance between Ogden, where my Mom, Dad, and brothers were, and Provo, where Rich's initial job was. Rich left his position to freelance as a speaking coach, but with the economy changing, his clientele quickly dried up, leaving us with little income.

While we had applied for SSI for Braden, who seemed most in need of a guaranteed income as he became an adult, we were still coming up far short of our bills month after month.

As all this was coming to a head, Rich had reconnected with a friend in Spokane who owned a house he no longer needed as a primary residence. He had suggested we bring the family up and house-sit while we got back on our feet financially. It wasn't the easiest decision, but in the end it offered the best solution to our current distress. So we packed up and moved back to Spokane. Ping Pong, anyone?

Once there, we decided to apply for disability on Rachel's behalf as well. With all of the issues surrounding her vision, large yearly doctor bills seemed a certainty for the rest of her life. Giving her the security of guaranteed healthcare was a logical step.

Between the move, the finances, the Social Security hoops, the insurance red tape, not to mention six kids and a husband in the house, life was threatening to completely overwhelm me. Even so, I remembered my promise after Brooklyn was born.

I knew that if I didn't stand up for my kids, no one would. I had been doing to my family, to my children, what had been done to me. Hiding from the fear of what NF could bring.

The time for fear was over. I needed to make sure my kids knew all about the health issues, all about NF, and all about how to stand up and take care of themselves.

I began to learn as much about Neurofibromatosis as possible. Out of necessity, I started educating the people around us: my children's teachers, my family and even the doctors that had been treating us for so long without ever bringing up NF as a significant issue. They needed to know what to look for and what to expect.

The more I learned, the more my guilt about passing this disorder on to my children began to take its toll. I was mad and frustrated, and I needed a way to vent my anger. I sat down at the computer and began a blog so negative Howard Stern would blush.

I entitled the blog "Life in the Big City" – but City started with SH and had two T's. My first post was about how much I hated NF, what it was doing to my body, and how ugly I felt. Honestly, for those moments of typing, it felt good, even freeing. But what good was it really doing? After reading the post to my husband, his response would begin a path that would change our lives forever.

"That's good hun," he said, a bit taken aback. "But have you ever thought about turning living with NF into something that inspires people?"

His words hit with a giant thud. What's he thinking, trying to go all motivational speaker on me? I resisted, and began to defend my actions. But then, as we bandied about less vulgar blog titles, the word THRIVE popped out. I almost fell out of my chair. "Thriving with NF"....what a concept!

I quickly created "Thriving with Neurofibromatosis" and started writing. My first blog post would introduce the new Kristi, both to my readers, and to myself. The new Thriving Girl. As I wrote, I made a very conscious effort to switch my thinking. Instead of hating NF, I began to think of ways to beat its cruelty.

It was a huge shift in my way of thinking, and my way of life. I was now creating something to live up to, something that had the potential to spread the word about NF worldwide. Not that day, but maybe someday.

That shift would prove to be vitally important, as the road ahead continued to lead me down one sharp turn after another.

Four months after our move, it was again time for Rachel's annual MRI. The first year was relatively easy. No questions, just compliance. But explaining an MRI to my now six-year-old proved much more challenging.

She was going to be anesthetized to keep her still, which would at least spare her from the jarring noise the apparatus makes as it scans the body. But what do I tell her is happening? Should I say she's going into suspended animation? A time machine? A giant tanning bed? In the end, I just gave it to her straight, and promised I would be by her side every second. She handled it all a lot better than I did.

As she closed her eyes and drifted off to sleep, I kissed her forehead gently, whispering "I love you," and slowly slipped away. I stopped halfway down the narrow walkway and leaned against a cold white wall. Sliding down, my face against my knees, just as I had been years before in my junior high locker room praying for myself, I prayed now for my precious Rachel. "Bless her Lord, keep her safe".

Lifting my head from my prayer, I then started to throw questions up to the universe. "Why? If God is powerful enough to separate oceans, and make a blind man see again, then why does He not cure this disorder that will ravage my child?" My questions worked me up into an intense anger. I was so mad at NF. My baby didn't deserve this! My body was hot, my jaw clenched, my hands tightly gripping the back of my neck.

Suddenly, an angelic woman in hospital scrubs touched my shoulder, "Mrs. Hopkins?"

I looked up at her, jolted out of my angry fog, my eyes red and teary, "Yes?"

"We're all done, she's just waking up in recovery - follow me." I slid up the wall and followed the nurse to the recovery area, where my baby girl was waiting. We smiled at each other from across the room.

"I have to tell you something really funny," the nurse insisted. "When your little girl woke up from anesthesia she was laughing so hard - she made the doctor and all the nurses laugh too."

My tension melted into grateful relief. I smiled and made my way across the room, taking my daughter in my arms. I hugged her for what seemed like an eternity. She gave me a tired grin, and asked for a purple popsicle. She had no real clue about the tests she just had, or the possible outcomes.

We sat in recovery for an hour and when given the okay to leave, we decided to skip the wheelchair taxi, and use the mommy piggy back instead! She climbed onto my back, and we galloped out of there. I didn't mind the lack of oxygen as her little arms choked tight my airway - I was just enjoying my time with my little Rachel Ray.

On the way home, we stopped to eat. I cherished the simplicity of our conversation: butterflies, rainbows, and how her favorite color used to be purple, but now it's blue! We took our time eating, pretending the french fries were people, giving them ketchup for lipstick. We put them together to kiss, and giggled like schoolgirls.

This is why I became a mother. Times like these I hold very close to heart. I want my kids to look back on their childhood and remember me as the mom that would stop the world for them. The bills can wait, the laundry can pile up, the dishes can stack. As long as I take the time to laugh with my kids, I can say I have had a great day. As we got up to go, I looked into her beautiful eyes, through her pink-rimmed glasses, and she looked right back at me.

"This is my most favoritest day ever," she declared.

"Mine too!" I replied.

Rachel's MRI results shocked me. It also explained many of the vision issues she'd been having, and possibly some of the behavior issues as well. They were concerned she had an Optic Glioma, but what they found instead was a narrowing of her optic pathways, and underdeveloped ventricles. The MRI also found a basal ganglia mass, which may have been interfering with her speech and motor skills.

After a visit to an ophthalmologist, we began patching her strong eye to force the weak eye to work harder, building muscle strength. Visual screenings every three months over the next year showed some progress being made, but it appears likely that Rachel will lose a significant percentage of her sight by adulthood.

In March of 2009, Braden started complaining of headaches. While I had taken the steps to have him officially diagnosed with NF, no MRI had been deemed 'medically necessary'. The migraines changed all that.

When I got the results on Braden's MRI, I talked to an on-call doctor who was clearly less than informed regarding NF.

Over the phone, he struggled reading through the complicated and confusing notes the technician left. He said the notes showed Braden having 'several' tumors at the base of his brain.

"What does 'several' mean?" I asked.

He responded that he didn't know, it wasn't charted. Just "There are many, Mrs. Hopkins."

He prescribed medicine for Braden's frequent headaches, and told me he would likely have to take it for the rest of his life. In addition, I was warned to pay close attention to his vision, and be sure he received regular eye checks. Physical and motor skills were also red-flagged for future observation.

"If he starts to get really clumsy, or falls down for no reason," the doctor said, "we need to have him in for another MRI."

This would be on top of the already required yearly MRI's. No optic nerve tumors were found and Braden's vision continues to be better than 20/20.

We decided to pull him from the 'mainstream' classroom, and placed him in a more one-on-one school environment. He was happier, and began retaining much more from the classroom than in previous years.

While his learning disabilities have been affecting Braden since pre-school, he is only now beginning to realize he's not like the other kids his age. His awareness helps him dismiss some of the tormenting from other kids, but works to tear down his self-esteem, while also giving him an excuse to not give his all to his schoolwork.

In addition to NF, he has been confirmed to have ADHD, and often seems unable to control himself, physically. He routinely rolls on the floor, hurls himself to the ground, and jumps from one spot to the next.

His attention span is almost non-existent, and pushing him to focus can put him in a dark mood. I find myself asking how much of this is simply being a teenager? How much is ADHD? How much is directly related to NF?

I walk a tightrope as a parent with him. He can be incredibly sweet and funny one moment, then angry, despondent, and defiant the next. Still, every time I look into his baby blue eyes, I see strength. Someone who won't let a diagnosis take him down. A kid who rocks at video games, who loves to take care of his baby sister, and a silly guy who, while often a bull in a china shop, knows how to make an entrance.

Balancing tolerance with discipline is my daily challenge with my oldest boy. But let's face it, we all face that challenge as parents to one degree or another.

Rachel and Braden both suffer NF and its effects on their lives with positive spirits, and seemingly boundless energy. If you met either of them, NF wouldn't even enter your mind.

They are an inspiration to me, and a confirmation to me that bringing NF out into the open was the best possible strategy.

I was going to have to follow their shining examples closely the next few months, because my road was about to get even darker at the next turn, Thriving or not.

CHAPTER 13
Donating Myself to Science

After my NF wake-up call with the obstetrician, my immediate focus was on the kids. I had to get them totally checked out and their problems dealt with. I wasn't afraid to investigate my own NF, but I admit I put it off by focusing on my kids first.

Sometimes I forget that one of the best things I can do for them is take care of me. *(Rich made me write this, because if it's in print, he says, he can always remind me.)*

When I mentioned my headaches to my new doctor in Spokane, I could put it off no longer.

She became only the second doctor in my adult life to notice Neurofibromatosis. Commenting on the "little bumps" on my neck and chest, she asked if I ever had an MRI. It was all I could do not to laugh. Of course not! I was too busy being overlooked, being a mom, and/or being broke to even consider an MRI in the past.

She was hesitant at first to order one and prescribed migraine medication instead. It was only when several different prescriptions failed to put a dent into the pain that I was finally allowed to get an MRI.

About a week after my MRI, as Rich and I were driving to pick up some groceries, the doctor called. Her profound accent made it difficult to understand what she was saying to me. I was diagnosed with Normal Pressure Hydrocephalus (NPH), enlarged ventricles and a M&M size brain tumor on my pituitary gland. I was also told that a small piece of my brain was coming down through my spinal opening.

The world started spinning around me. "Did I just hear this right?" I laid the cell phone in my lap, Rich looking over at me anticipating the news. I couldn't speak. Rich pulled to the roadside and held my hands. I'm sure he knew from the look in my eyes the news wasn't good.

I felt like I had been run over by a truck. Meeting with a neurologist, and subsequently a neurosurgeon offered me no solutions, no answers. I sat across from these doctors as they told me that a shunt, which my brother Mike had successfully been using to offset hydrocephalus for most of his life, wasn't guaranteed to work for me, and might make things worse.

I was told, ironically enough, that I most likely had been suffering from excess liquid around my brain since childhood, and had compensated for it well. I don't know how they can consider daily headaches, and far too frequent migraines, 'compensating'. If doctors had paid more attention to me as a child, I might have had a shunt put in 20 years ago, saving years of pain. Now they're telling me it's too late?

My brain tumor is called a Lipoma, and again, nothing can be safely done. I felt I would've been better off not having the MRI at all. Knowing only made things worse, especially if no one would fix the problems, for fear of causing bigger ones. I refused to go back to my neurologist after she essentially told me I was exaggerating the pain I was having. She told me that people with Neurofibromatosis do not experience this kind of pain.

"Stick with the migraine medication and see me in six months," she coldly blurted out.

"Yeah - I don't think so!" I wanted to say, but held my tongue.

Frustrated and angry, I wanted crawl back into my hole. Certainly hiding was much better than having to face this ridiculous reality. I may have successfully stood up for my kids, but personally, I was getting nowhere.

Before my Thriving declaration, I would have just sucked it up and pushed the pain under all the concerns of the rest of my life. Now, I owed it to myself, my family, and in a way, to anyone whoever came upon my blog, to search for other ways to get help.

That search led me to the home page of the National Institutes of Health (NIH) in Maryland. I was looking for open studies to participate in, and suddenly there it was, a study about Neurofibromatosis. I immediately applied, and to my surprise, got a call back just a week later.

It was a study about variability, especially with individuals who are affected by NF within families. I immediately thought of me and Mike. Who more perfect to participate in this study than a brother and sister affected by NF in severely different ways?

During the phone call, I talked about life with NF and brought up my brother. With Mike in Utah and me in Washington, it was tricky working out the details, but by mid-July, the trip was set. I took a connecting flight through Salt Lake City, and met up with Mike.

Dad, his wife Pat, and Pop, my dad's dad, came out to see us both off. I was shocked to see Pop in a wheelchair. Just months before he was as I always saw him - tall and strong, a jovial soul who loved to greet me with giant bear hugs. The man at the airport was just a shell of his former self, looking frail and tired.

Still, I could still see the glint in Pop's eyes as I leaned over to hug him before Mike and I headed towards security. Just weeks later, Pop passed away. I was unable to attend the funeral, but I was grateful for the opportunity to see him, if only for a few short minutes.

Once Mike and I arrived in Bethesda, it seemed like we'd taken a time machine back to the '80s. The Bonnie and Clyde duo rides again! We checked into a surprisingly nice hotel and headed out to grab a bite to eat. Just around the corner from the hotel was a little burger place where Mike and I ordered greasy french fries and two ginormous hamburgers.

Just like we did as kids in California, we stuffed our faces, made fun of each other, and laughed at our own pitifully bad jokes. It didn't matter we were now adults, both squarely facing the uncertainty of NF for the next week. Tonight, we were just brother and sister, shutting out the world.

We had to catch a bus to NIH, and when we got there, I couldn't believe how huge it was. The levels of security alone were enough to think I was about to enter Fort Knox. They gave us ID badges, and, just like the airport, we went through a body scanner before heading inside.

It didn't take long for the doctors to order labs and start sending us around the building for tests. Finding our way around NIH took some practice, and it was easy to take a wrong turn. Mike and were supposed to be headed toward the Phlebotomy Lab, and were getting turned around. We entered yet another wrong room, and I asked Mike to go over to the security guard and ask where we needed to be.

Mike, half deaf after his bicycle accident, had to ask me to repeat myself. Suddenly, my little sister instincts took over, and I whispered into Mikey's ear for him to go ask the front desk where he needed to go for a - *lobotomy*.

Mike approached the guard and asked the question in his deep and relatively loud tone of voice, just as I'd instructed. The room fell silent. I hid behind my magazine, failing miserably to muffle my giggles. Unable to hold back, I erupted into enormous laughter. The security guard did a double take, and Mikey just stood there, the perfect straight man. He laughed it off once he realized what his evil ol' sis had done. Mike – you are, and always have been, a great guy!

That week, we were both examined head to toe, and asked to talk about all that NF has brought to, and taken away from, our lives. For me, it was the first time I could finally share the pain, the headaches, blurry vision, back pain, the finger pain, with someone who didn't just believe me, but actually understood.

For Mike, it was more complicated. He talked to the doctors about the tumor that had deformed his face. We were impressed that they wanted to know more, as doctors back home had not attempted to address the issue. At first they thought the mass had more to do with an infected or swollen saliva gland, but it turned out to be an NF-related tumor.

At the dental clinic, Mike was afraid and embarrassed about what they would find. NF can cause severe dental erosion, and Mike had reached a point of no return with most of his teeth. I tried to talk to him and reassure him. They did find major dental problems, but he was treated with caring hands and deserved respect.

When Mike returned to Utah, he followed through with the referrals he was given, and both the facial tumor and eroding teeth were dealt with in short order.

Getting so much attention was a first for me. I was excited and uncomfortable at the same time. Finally, my NF was being acknowledged, but more than that, it was being accepted and treated. I started getting answers to questions I had been holding back my entire life.

When I asked about the pain in my fingers, Dr. Stewart arranged an MRI. The images revealed tumors that piqued his interest, and the interest of other doctors working directly with glomus tumors. I had never heard of these before, but NIH had, and asked if I'd like to have them removed.

Wow. I had been having the pain in my fingertips for as long as I can remember, and now I didn't just have answers, I had a potential solution. I told them I'd have to think about whether I'd be able to make it back for surgery, but truthfully, I didn't have to think long!

The doctors at NIH seemed to truly care about the people in their study. We were not just numbers, just a series of test results. I finally felt I'd found a place that understood everything I had been trying to say for so many years. NIH is an oasis, populated by people who actually speak my language.

I came home more positive than I'd been in years. The fact that Rich had managed to keep all the kids fed and alive during the week I was gone topped off what had been a truly miraculous time in my life.

And for the first time, life was beginning to get better, instead of worse, with each passing day.

CHAPTER 14
NF Girls Gone Wild!

Following my experience with NIH, my attitude towards NF continued to transform. Yes, I still hated it, but instead of giving it the cold shoulder, I confronted it every way I could.

With Rich's help, I created a line of Thrivewear, with slogans declaring "Thriving with NF", "I (heart) someone with NF", and even put an NF spin on all those bumper stickers such as "Firemen like it HOT" - creating "NFer's Like it Bumpy"!

Hiding NF wasn't going to help anyone - if announcing it on clothes and coffee mugs could increase awareness, why not?

I went ahead and scheduled my return trip to NIH, thrilled to have the chance to have pain-free hands. My new year would start off with a week back in Maryland.

In the meantime, I began searching out opportunities to spread the word about NF, and raise money for research on new treatments, perhaps even a preventative cure. I felt emancipated, and it was out of my new-found excitement the idea for this book was born.

One opportunity came by way of Facebook: a makeover project in Northwest Woman, a magazine Rich had briefly worked for. I sent in my application, and was chosen to share my challenges with its readers, as well as my new look.

Ironically, it almost didn't happen, as the first makeover artist scheduled for me was scared off when we he found out about my NF. He was afraid others in his studio would 'catch it', or his students would be uncomfortable working on me. Despite my attempts to educate him on NF, he declined my makeover.

The magazine's publisher, however, didn't give up, and found another studio in town who had no problem taking on the assignment. It is amazing that even in this age of instant information, ignorance can still be rampant.

I also contacted the local Make-A-Wish Foundation, intent on volunteering. Unbeknownst to me, they were checking me out after I had mentioned my family's experiences with NF on our first phone call. Me, and my kids.

They had gone to my blog, and read several posts about Rachel and her vision challenges. They surprised me, telling me Neurofibromatosis was a qualifying condition for a Wish, and suggested I apply for one on Rachel's behalf.

When they asked me what Rachel was most interested in, I told them how much she loved the Disney Princesses, and they let me know that trips to Disney World were one of their most popular wishes. If Rachel asked, there was a good chance her wish could come true. Never in a million years had I considered this a possibility. I sent in the application, but said nothing to Rachel.

My date of departure for NIH drew near, and life threw us another curve ball. Rich unexpectedly ended up with a job that would again send him traveling, and he would be gone the last two days of my surgical visit.

My first thoughts, though, were not "Great – it figures I'd lose this chance," or to complain to God, as it might have been just a year before. Instead, I chose to believe I would be going regardless, and we would somehow find someone to care for our six kids during those two days.

Thankfully, Rich's mom, despite her trepidation, took time out from her job, and normally sedate lifestyle, to help. When I arrived home, the kids were happy and safe, and my mother-in-law had even managed to avoid being tied to a chair by her six crazy grandkids.

My second adventure at NIH seemed a bit scarier without my brother at my side. That fear quickly faded when I spent my first night completely alone in a quiet hotel room. For a mom of six, you must understand, this was a bit like winning the Powerball Lotto. I had never slept so soundly. I went to bed early, knowing I had to get to NIH at oh-dark-hundred to prep for surgery.

When I arrived, it was time to hurry up and wait. Life happens, as they say, and my surgery was delayed until the next day. I was a bit worried my stay might be extended, creating more problems with Rich leaving, but he assured me that no matter what, all would be taken care of at home.

I believe the delay was meant to be, because I was soon checked into a room with a woman who was also staying a week, with the same challenges I was experiencing. At that point in my life, I had not met anyone other than my family that was affected by NF. She was a mom, like me, and was also determined not to let her disorder keep her and her family from living the life they wanted.

She helped get me mentally ready for the surgery, telling me what to expect, since she had the same surgery a few months before. The removal of my glomus tumors was one of the best things I could have done. The surgery consisted of removing my fingernails, then scooping the tumor out. A few stitches later and I was back in my room to recover, my hand bandaged up like a mummy. I could immediately feel the difference.

My new best friend helped me forget about the pain by finding endless ways to make me laugh. She just had a way of looking at life that was fun, lighthearted, and often downright comical. She suggested we walk around the hospital topless, to give everyone an up-close and personal lesson in what having Neurofibromatosis was.

"Wooo-hooooo! NF Girls Gone Wild!" I said, my Krazy Kristi side starting to wake up a bit. This time though, I managed to avoid the temptation. I had no desire to again be caught in that state of undress. I wasn't in high school anymore!

Even without streaking down the hallways, we became known as the 'class clowns' of the hospital floor. Cracking wise about the good-looking doctors, playing jokes on the nurses, and sharing private laughs that must have left the staff wondering if we should be transferred to a more secure wing, we made the most of our moments in the sun.

Leaving was bittersweet. I couldn't wait to see my kids, but I also knew I was returning to a world ignorant about NF. I was wishing I could just move my family right there on hospital grounds, safe from the judgments that come with having a disorder few knew about, and even fewer understood.

Rich's new job not only meant that he would be traveling for most of the year, but that we would again be moving. Penske, if you're looking for a spokesperson, I am your ultimate Mother Trucker. I've logged more hours behind the steering wheel of a moving truck than Lindsay Lohan has spent in front of a judge.

This time, our destination was Denver, Colorado, and this time, I was pumped. Rich and I had been wanting to find our way to Denver for years. He had many friends from his days living there after college with whom he had kept in touch.

My memories of the beauty of Colorado from my time there years before were vivid, and the thought of moving somewhere because I wanted to, instead of being forced to, made me feel wonderful.

In mid-December, before we even knew this job was available, I had even put a picture of a house in Denver up on our 'dream board', despite my knee-jerk resistance to motivational tactics and Law of Attraction mumbo-jumbo. We didn't even know the job existed at the time, so maybe all that mumbo-jumbo really works. At the very least, it proved that God will make things happen if you let Him know what you want.

Rich and I decided we weren't going to move until the end of the school year, both to see if the job was going to work out, and to give our kids some stability. Riley, who was finishing up third grade, complained to us that she never spent a full year at one school – staying in Spokane a few extra months was the least we could do.

Growing up, I swore I'd never let what happened to me happen to my kids. I found myself suddenly understanding what my dad faced, moving every year. Divorces, financial challenges, job changes – sometimes life just doesn't go according to plan.

CHAPTER 15
What, Me Worry?

Just a few weeks after returning from NIH, the Make-A-Wish team came out to meet with my little princess. A month later, she found out her wish was granted - the entire family would be flying to Orlando in March!

But even as this good news was exciting the family, NF took another swing at us, and my Thriving attitude. Bailey began to complain about dizziness and headaches. Of all the kids, she had shown the fewest effects of NF, other than her academic challenges. She had not had any further medical follow up. Once again, I found myself taking a child in for an MRI.

Three days later, I got a call from a neurosurgeon's office asking me to make an appointment. Right away, I knew something was wrong. With Rachel and Braden, the pediatrician called me to notify me of the results, without much urgency. Now a neurosurgeon was on the case?

I panicked and began asking questions to the nurse on the phone about what was found. She couldn't answer me, and I became more scared for Bailey. Waiting a week for the appointment day to arrive seemed like waiting an eternity. Seven days later, I was impatiently sitting at the doctor's office waiting to discuss Bailey's MRI results. I thumbed through a magazine, peeking every now and then to my kids, who were playing quite nicely in the nook across from me. My nerves were shot. All I could do was close my eyes and pray that the news today would be good news.

The nurse called Bailey's name and we all headed back into the exam room. Brooklyn and Riker slid their hands along the wall and jumped to avoid the cracks in the floor.

"You okay Mom?" Bailey asks.

"I'm just thinking about you, sweetie."

She puts her arm around my shoulders and says, "Well, I hope you're not worried. I mean what's to worry about?"

Bailey amazes me everyday. She struggles in school, has very few friends, and seems to spend much of her day in a quiet, brooding state. Still, she always has this way of comforting me when I should be comforting her, and looking at the brightest side of the darkest times.

"I know everything is going to be okay, no matter what!" she continued to reassure me.

She walked confidently into the room, and was asked to sit up on the table. Brooklyn and Riker headed for the chairs at the window sill. I stood and answered a few questions, making sure we got a full history in Bailey's chart.

"How was your pregnancy with her?"
"When was Bailey diagnosed with NF?"
"What are the symptoms that Bailey is experiencing?"

Answering all these questions made me feel uncomfortable, but I knew it was important. "Thrive," I kept repeating my mantra in my head, "Thrive."

The doctor came in and sat down next to me. We talked about the tumor that was found in Bailey's brain, and he assured me that this was a slow-growing, benign tumor. Still, I began to feel an overwhelming sense of guilt well up inside.

Bailey hopped down from the table and slid into the chair next to me. She saw the worry in my eyes, and she understood that even though this was a benign tumor, it was still very serious. She held my hand and whispered, "I love you Mommy, I'm going to be okay!"

The doctor smiled at this and raised his eyebrows, as if to say, "WOW, I'm impressed!" I smiled too.

He told us about the placement of the tumor, and all the possible effects that had already occurred, and what could happen next.

"Bailey's hearing could be impaired and since this tumor is right on a nerve that controls facial muscles, her face could become deformed," he explained. Bailey squeezed my hand tight.

We had two possible treatments to consider. First, we could watch and wait. If the tumor wasn't getting larger at a fast rate, surgery might prove a rash decision. Second, instead of waiting for changes in the tumor and risking greater damage, schedule immediate surgery to remove the tumor. We were squarely between a rock and a hard place.

The choice wouldn't be solely ours, however. He was assembling a team of doctors and they would contact us about what they felt was the best approach. The doctor looked at me and put his hands on my shoulder. "We have time, this is not imminent," he assured me.

But I wanted to do something *right now*!

"I HATE NEUROFIBROMATOSIS!" The scream echoed through my brain, but I kept it off my lips.

When we received a picture of Bailey's MRI, she said "That's soooooooo cool!" She immediately pointed at the tumor and asked, "Is that it?"

"Yes" I replied.

She stuck her tongue at the image and said, "We're gonna get you, sucka!" I just laughed, and stuck my tongue out at the tumor too.

As we left the office, Bailey looked over at me. "I can't wait to get home and blog about this, because I'm not afraid, and I want to let everyone know that I'm not afraid!"

Over the weekend I saw Bailey looking rather distracted and lost in thought. "What are you thinking about honey?"

"Oh just about my tumor and the hospital." she replied. I went over to her and sat down, asking her if she had any questions. I told her to try not to worry about this.

She looks up at me and bluntly says, "I didn't say I was worried - I'm just thinking about it. Will I get to stay in a hospital? Will I get to stay overnight? I'm actually excited to do something about this. What are we waiting for!?"

I just hugged her. "You're so awesome Bailey, I love you!"

CHAPTER 16
When You Wish Upon a Star

The build up and anticipation for the fulfillment of Rachel's Wish was tremendous. The kids made a countdown chart, and each day we crossed off the days until we left. The excitement reached a fevered pitch when the kids could count the days left on their fingers!

Rich took a week off and came home to a living room full of suitcases Make-A-Wish had purchased for us. He kept us on schedule – we had to leave early the very next day, and sleep was essential if we were going to safely and sanely escort six kids through three airports and three thousand miles.

From the airport in Orlando, we headed straight to Give Kids the World Village. It was more amazing in person than their website could describe. The bright colors and kid-friendly shapes of the buildings were made even brighter by the warm, caring staff inside. It was just what Rachel, and our family, needed!

Even though plane delays and layovers got us to Orlando late in the evening, we were quickly welcomed and checked in. A stuffed Mickey for Rachel, toys for her brothers and sisters, and T-shirts for everyone were passed out. Dinner was waiting, saved for us by Katie's Kitchen, their on-site take-out window, sponsored by Boston Chicken.

The next morning, we were off to Walt Disney World. As the monorail approached the park, Rachel saw the beautiful castle in the distance, her eyes lighting up. "Is that Cinderella's castle, Mama?" she asked, anticipating what may be hiding beyond the enormous doors.

Rachel's wish came true as she headed up the back hall of the 'Meet the Princesses' area, and was escorted to the front of the line. Cinderella, Sleeping Beauty, and Belle from *Beauty and the Beast* were all there, ready to hug Rachel and her sisters.

She was able to talk to each one of them, while the park photographer snapped pictures. Braden and Riker, typical boys, not wanting any part of it, hid behind the trashcans. Belle, however, sneaked over to plant a quick kiss on Braden's cheek. I've never seen him blush so much in his life!

Rachel skipped out of the castle with her autograph book in hand, so happy and carefree. For that moment, there was no NF. Brain tumors didn't exist, and pain was the furthest thing from our minds. We were living in a fairy tale, where wishes were reality.

We spent two days exploring the Magic Kingdom, and two days at the Universal Studio Parks. It was great to have a truly worry-free week, even one that found us screaming on one roller coaster ride after another.

Each night, we'd return to our villa, where Village staff would leave gifts of games, snacks, and movies for the kids. We ate most nights at the Kitchen, but also enjoyed the Gingerbread House, a sit down buffet-style restaurant sponsored by Perkin's, where we talked with many of the other guests.

The final day, we stayed 'home', exploring the village's putt putt course, riding the beautiful merry-go-round at least a million times, and, at the kids insistence, swimming in one of the outdoor pools near our villa.

Mickey, Minnie, and Goofy all showed up at the Village theatre, and posed for pictures. It was a fun and semi-peaceful way to rest up from the events of the week, in preparation to head home the next day.

Give Kids the World is truly magical. From the moment you enter the gates, it's like the world transforms around you. Every single person inside these gates knows what it's like to cry for a child who is suffering. There is an overwhelming web of emotions there, but what I did not feel was sorrow, or sadness, instead I felt a great deal of thankfulness.

Walking into the Castle of Miracles, seeing the ceiling of stars inscribed with names of past visitors pulled out many, many tears from me, as I knew that many, probably most, of those names were truly stars in heaven.

Rachel being a part of this building individualized each and every one of these stars for me. I was humbled to be here, and grateful that Rachel wasn't facing a terminal disease.

Thankful she still was given this opportunity to see her dream in bright, living color, before, if NF has its way, her world fades to black.

The very existence of a place like this, for families to be able to come together and share in their child's wishes in the midst of their obstacles, is the biggest fulfilled wish of all.

When it was time to check out of the Village, Rachel began to cry. "I don't want to leave this place Mama. I feel good when I'm here!"

I just hugged her. "So do I, Ray. So do I."

I reminded Rachel about her star, how a part of her will forever be a part of this Village - and the Village will forever be a part of her.

She smiled, and together, we headed home.

CHAPTER 17
Thriving in Denver

With Orlando behind us, Denver now lay before us in three short months. Rich spent most of his time away on the job, coming back just a day before packing the truck and making the two-day drive.

Once in Denver, the process of finding doctors and securing insurance began. I had spent some time researching the Denver area, and was excited to have access to the Children's Hospital in Aurora, just 30 minutes or so from where we lived.

I also got in touch with the Denver Chapter of CTF, arranged to be part of a local NF Walk, and attended a NF symposium. Even with Rich back out on the road, the church he had been attending welcomed me and the kids with open arms. Being alone with six kids in a new city was made much easier by my new support system.

Just a week after arriving in Denver, I put Bailey on a plane to Salt Lake City, for a week-long NF Camp she had been given a scholarship to attend.

At the airport we ran into Philip, a boy with NF who appeared on MTV's True Life episode focusing on NF. He was headed to camp as well, and he and Bailey made fast friends.

It was tough on me to let her go for a week, but I knew she'd have a blast. The camp had created a packed schedule to keep them entertained, and Bailey would finally have a chance to find out more about both NF, and herself. She came back with a bigger smile, a healthy dose of self-confidence, and I swear, an extra inch of height. I always hoped my daughter would look up to me, and now I was looking up to her!

Once she returned, it was time again to focus on Bailey's tumor. The move had put us in a frustrating position. The doctors in Spokane recommended we go ahead with the surgery, but we wouldn't be able to schedule early enough for them to provide aftercare, which left the doctors uncomfortable.

If we waited until we were in Denver, the insurance would lapse, leaving us with tens of thousands of dollars in doctor bills. Bailey and the other kids remained on state insurance, in part because even with the new job, we couldn't afford the insurance they offered, and we were still making so little money that we easily met state requirements.

Rich assured me that if surgery were absolutely necessary, we would bear the debt. Before that step was taken, we ended up getting Bailey qualified for SSI, and she was able to visit Denver's Children's Hospital earlier than we expected to get checked out.

Unlike Spokane, Denver has many doctors that understand NF, and a few who actually specialize in it. At our appointment, a team came in to examine Bailey and were enthusiastic, from a medical point of view, about her case.

We had brought a CD with the MRI scan on it, and left it in the doctor's hands. We fully expected to go through with surgery, as the doctors in Spokane had suggested. To our surprise, word came back to watch and wait. I was infuriated. Watch and wait? For what? For the tumor to do more damage?

The doctor reasoned that the tumor might take years to grow large enough to do damage, and assured me we would keep a close eye on it. I was still frustrated. Waiting leaves me helpless. What mother wants to be helpless when it comes to their child?

In the next few months, we'll go in and have another look. Until then, we wait – and we Thrive anyway.

(Editor's Note: Since the first printing of Thriving with Neurofibromatosis, Bailey has been diagnosed with a non-cancerous, but growing, brain tumor, and is undergoing chemotherapy. Ironically, NF may have saved her life by providing a reason for regular MRI's. Without them, this tumor may not have been discovered until it had grown far too large for effective treatment.)

A Thriving Life

This, my friends, is my story. At least my story up to now. While this is the end of the book, it is still only the beginning of My Thriving Life.

If you picked up this book thinking it was going to be filled with all positive, Tony Robbins rah-rah, be all you can be hyperbole, well – Surprise! I do positive, I just do it in my own way. It has taken me a long time to get here, and I get up everyday reminding myself to be thankful, to be strong, and to Thrive.

As I examine my last 36 years through the lens of NF, I'm surprised by how much fun I had even when life seemed to be crumbling around me. I credit my parents for doing the best job they could with the information they had at the time.

While I may have had my unhappy moments, overall, I am blessed by a mom and dad who truly care about me and my six kids.

Writing this book has shown me how I am truly a product of my past. Both my weaknesses and strengths were initially forged in the fires of a disconnected, and sometimes dysfunctional, youth.

No matter how hard I wished to hide, it was inevitable that I would eventually fight back. The way I fight back, however, is truly a result of who I have become over the last three years, and the people in my life who have supported and encouraged me along the way, both directly and indirectly. Sometimes it's the people who anger us the most who push us to do what we never thought we could.

The last thing I ever thought I would do would be to shout to the world about Neurofibromatosis. I spent the first 33 years of my life doing exactly the opposite. I did everything I could to hide from the world, hide my disorder, and hide myself. I lived each day in deep denial. I accept that. Now I am taking responsibility for it.

It took me facing the reality that my children were going to be affected by NF whether I accepted it or not to begin to deal with this progressive, life-long disorder. I didn't like it, I didn't want it, and I didn't think it was fair - but it was real, nonetheless.

Once I began to break down the walls of denial, and built up some power to fight back, I went beyond accepting it, and started embracing it. As the old saying goes, I have NF, but it doesn't have me. The tighter I hold it, the less power it has over me.

I admit, I still get angry, I still get depressed. But I am learning to use that energy - to turn it into something good. Whether it's writing in my blog, creating Thriving with NF bracelets, or finding ways to work within the NF community, I am determined to gain greater awareness for our disorder, and greater acceptance from a world who still thinks NF is the Elephant Man's disease.

If you're reading this, and you have NF, how are you dealing with it from day to day? It's not easy, certainly, and I realize there are many who suffer from NF to a much greater degree than me or any of my family.

Perhaps you don't have NF, but hoped to understand those around you that do. Do your NF friend a favor, and hand this book to them. I hope there are many doctors reading this. You need to understand how we feel to be able to fully treat us and help us face our challenging road. Share this book with your staff – please.

My prayer for the NF community is that, together, we realize a Thriving Life is possible. A genetic disorder, whether it's Neurofibromatosis, Muscular Dystrophy, Cystic Fibrosis, Multiple Sclerosis or any of a hundred others, does not need to limit you, your potential, or your happiness while you still have the ability to choose your thoughts and actions.

My story is just that, my story. What's yours? It doesn't have to be the same tomorrow that it was yesterday, or today.

What the future will bring for me and my family, and our lives with NF, is uncertain. All I know for sure is that my responsibility to my kids, to the NF community, and to myself, is to continue to Thrive. To educate myself, to take command of my attitude, to share my story with others, and to yield to the perfection that God created within me.

I hope you found some hope, a dash of inspiration, and maybe a laugh or two as you read Thriving with NF: Kristi's Story. As you put this book down and head back into the world, remember this – I never thought I would Thrive with Neurofibromatosis. Until I did.

Thrive On!

The E.A.S.Y.
Way to Thrive

EDUCATION - Educate yourself about Neurofibromatosis. Fear breeds inside the unknown, and ignorance leads nowhere. Research what is known about NF, and find other people to share notes with. New information is discovered about NF every year, and research continues to create new advances in treatment. The more you know, the more you'll know how to Thrive.

ATTITUDE & ACTION - Live, think and breathe a Thriving Attitude. Who are you when no one is watching? Who are you when EVERYONE is watching? Your attitude will affect your actions, and your actions will certainly affect your attitude, and impact your ability to Thrive On. William Glasser says it well: "If you want to change your attitude, start with a change in behavior." Participate in research. Contact, or if necessary, start, your local NF chapter. Speak, and let the world hear your story.

SHARE - When faced with ignorance or judgment, do not turn away, Share. Share who you are and what you live with every day. Share lovingly with the child that points in your direction. Share respectfully with doctors who need to understand more about you and your life. Share openly with each other, so we know we're not alone.

YIELD – Yield to the possibility that you can be whoever you choose to be. We are our own worst enemies when we choose to believe all the world tells us about ourselves. When we believe we are defective, deformed, and depressed, instead of powerful, perfect people who deserve respect and love, we fail ourselves, our world and our creator. As Gandhi said so profoundly: *"Be the change you want to see in the world."*

Go out and live a bold and confident life – and don't let the world convince you you deserve anything less.

Thrive On!

Resources

Thriving with Neurofibromatosis
www.thrivingwithnf.com

National Institute of Health
9000 Rockville Pike
Bethesda, Maryland 20892
www.nih.gov

Children's Tumor Foundation
95 Pine Street, 16th Floor
New York, N.Y. 10005-4002
www.ctf.org

Make -A-Wish Foundation
4742 N. 24th St., Suite 400
Phoenix, AZ 85016-4862
www.wish.org

Give Kids the World
210 South Bass Road
Kissimmee, FL 34746
www.gktw.org

About the Author

Kristi Hopkins is a mother to six wonderful children, three of whom share her genetic disorder of Neurofibromatosis. Her many talents include cartooning, scrapbooking, cake decorating, making diaper cakes, writing, and maintaining her sanity.

After spending the majority of her youth in Southern California, Kristi now resides in Broomfield, CO. When she's not managing the household, she's actively working to let the world know more about Neurofibromatosis.

Kristi's blog, *http://thrivingwithneurofibromatosis.blogspot.com* has been the cornerstone of her passion for evangelizing on behalf of NFer's around the world since she started it in 2009.

Kristi welcomes the opportunity to speak to your group about Thriving with Neurofibromatosis. Contact her at Kristi.Hopkins@gmail.com for details on how to book her at your next event.

DISCARD

Made in the USA
Charleston, SC
18 September 2013

NOV -- 2013

330 8889